THE PHYSIOLOGY OF THE JOINTS

Seventh edition

A.I. KAPANDJI

Honorary Member of the French Society of Orthopaedics and Traumatology
Honorary Member and President (1987-1988) of the French Society of Hand Surgeons
Member of the American Society for Surgery of the Hand and of the Italian Society for Surgery of the Hand
Corresponding Foreign Member of the Argentine Society of Orthopaedics and Traumatology

THE PHYSIOLOGY OF THE JOINTS

Foreword by Professor Gérard Saillant and Professor Robert Merle d'Aubigné

3

Seventh edition

1. A Global View of the Spinal Column
2. The Pelvic Girdle
3. The Lumbar Spine
4. The Thoracic Spine and the Thorax
5. The Cervical Spine
6. The Head

539 original drawings by the author
Translated by Dr Louis Honoré

HANDSPRING
PUBLISHING

Handspring Publishing
Carmelite House
50 Victoria Embankment
London EC4Y 0DZ
www.handspringpublishing.com

Seventh edition first published in 2018 in French by Éditions Maloine under the title
Anatomie fonctionnelle: 3. Tête et rachis by A.I. Kapandji.
Copyright © Éditions Maloine 2018 – ISBN: 978-2-224-03542-6

Seventh edition first published in 2019 in English in the United Kingdom by Handspring Publishing (an imprint of Jessica Kingsley Publishers, an imprint of Hodder & Stoughton Ltd, an Hachette UK Company) by arrangement with Éditions Maloine.

ISBN 978-1-912085-61-3

British Library Cataloguing in Publication Data

A catalogue record for this book is available from the British Library

Library of Congress Cataloguing in Publication Data

A catalogue record for this book is available from the Library of Congress

Notice
Neither the Publisher nor the Author assume any responsibility for any loss or injury and/or damage to persons or property arising out of or relating to any use of the material contained in this book. It is the responsibility of the treating practitioner, relying on independent expertise and knowledge of the patient, to determine the best treatment and method of application for the patient.

Cover painting: A.I. Kapandji

Printed in France

To my wife
To my artist mother
To my surgeon father
To my maternal grandfather

Foreword to the fifth edition

The physiology of the spine cannot be said to be easy even for surgeons who specialize in locomotor problems. Someone with a feeling for mechanics, an affinity for precision, an ability to see things three-dimensionally had to feel a vocation for this work – and that person had to be an able teacher with a gift for simplifying complex ideas. Such are the qualities of Adalbert Kapandji, who has put into this work his great artistic talent along with his sense of precision and of beauty, all of which have resulted in a most inventive layout. We all learned anatomy from diagrams, but they were flat and fixed, whereas with his cut-out models Dr Kapandji has created the three-dimensional diagram.

The task of teaching the spine used to be more difficult, since its complex movements are harder to understand and explain. Dr Kapandji's achievement, which was already outstanding in the first two volumes, is even more striking in the volume it is my privilege to introduce.

In my opinion his success is complete. I envy young surgeons who have such a book available to them. I have no doubt that, in making the understanding of the mechanics of the spine easier and in explaining the forces that cause deformities, this book contributes enormously to the very important progress that is being made and will continue to be made in the treatment of spinal lesions.

Professor R. MERLE D'AUBIGNÉ

Foreword to the sixth edition

The spine is no longer an anatomical mystery now that its challenging physiology has been explained in this book. Despite the variations peculiar to its various segments – cervical, thoracic, lumbar and sacral – the structural and functional principles remain identical whatever the segment. Its physiology is actually simple and logical, yet how many foolish things have been said and written about and done to the spine!

Everything seems simple when it becomes clear that protection of the neural axis must be assured, along with a careful balance between the two principal functions of the spine: stability and mobility. Crowning the vertebral column is the head, which plays a social and relational role inasmuch as it is the seat of the five senses, of which four are directly connected to the brain.

The triumph of Adalbert Kapandji is to have shown all this simply and naturally by means of a clear, understandable text enlivened by extraordinarily simple diagrams and colour drawings. In this book everything seems perfectly simple – if only someone had thought of it like this before – and the myth of a complicated spinal column naturally fades away.

Further expanded in its sixth edition, this thought-provoking reference book, with its exciting subject and extraordinary layout, both didactic and enchanting, will be avidly read. So it will be useful, or rather essential, equally for medical students and for any practitioner interested in the locomotor apparatus: orthopaedists, rheumatologists, physicians, neurosurgeons, physiotherapists, osteopaths and even musicians and top-level athletes interested in understanding the workings of their own bodies.

Adalbert I. Kapandji deserves heartfelt thanks for having taken us back so enjoyably to certain basic facts.

Professor G. SAILLANT
Member of the Academy of Surgery;
Former Dean of the Faculty of Medicine at Pitié Salpêtrière (Paris VI);
Former Head of Orthopaedics at the Pitié Salpêtrière Hospital.

Note on the sixth edition

This new edition of volume 3 of *The Physiology of the Joints* follows the lead of volume 1: not only have all the plates been redone in colour but new ones have been added as well as some new pages, and in consequence the text has been entirely recast. The anatomical terms follow international nomenclature. The original chapters have been enriched: for example, the chapter on the cervical spine contains the addition of a page on the vertebral artery, which is so closely linked to the vertebrae that it is highly susceptible to damage from clumsy manipulation. Important knowledge about the vertebral pedicle has led to great advances in spinal surgery, thanks to the introduction of the pedicular screw. In the chapter on the lumbar spine, different physical postures adopted in everyday and professional life are investigated. Some new chapters have been added, as for example the chapter dealing with the pelvis and describing the role of the perineum in the physiological activities of urination, defecation, erection and labour and delivery. A chapter on the head introduces for the first time a description of the physiology of the temporomandibular joint, so essential in feeding. We learn too that the movements of the eyeballs are those of a perfect enarthrosis, and this ideal spherical joint, comparable to others of the same type, like the hip and the shoulder, must obey the same rules of mechanics. The physiology of the oblique muscles is explained in terms of the pathetic facial expression. All this is illustrated with new original drawings. Overall, this sixth edition of volume 3, like that of volume 1 (and the future volume 2) is really a completely new book, both in layout and content, and consequently deserves renewed attention from readers interested in the biomechanics of the human body.

Note on the seventh edition

The first edition of this work was published in the sixties, and since then it has been popular not only in France but also abroad with translations into fourteen languages. This seventh edition is a celebration of a new approach to the teaching of the functional anatomy of the human body and of biomechanics in general.

We have done our best to improve this book and to add new ideas using appendices devoted to the concepts of mass, weight, barycentre, joint hypermobility and the law of parsimony.

The end of this book still features the traditional mechanical models unique to it. These can be viewed as practical challenges in biomechanics to students who will have the courage and the patience to build them; they will thus experience manually the difficulties encountered in creating some well-balanced joints.

Contents

Chapter 5 – THE CERVICAL SPINE.. 186

Chapter 1

A GLOBAL VIEW OF THE SPINAL COLUMN

The human species belongs to the subphylum Vertebrata and represents the final stage of a long evolution that started with fish after they left the sea to colonize the land.

Its locomotor system, centred on the spinal column, or the spine, is the result of the transformation of a prototype already recognizable in the crossopterygians, which were four-legged and caudate animals intermediate between fish and reptiles. All the components of this original model are still present in humans with some modifications, notably these two:

* the loss of the tail
* the transition to the erect position.

These changes have wrought profound alterations in the axis of the human body (i.e. the spinal column), which nonetheless is still made up of short bones stacked one on top of another and still able to move freely among themselves (i.e. the vertebrae). This osteoarticular complex not only supports the body but also protects the spinal cord, a veritable message-transmitting cable linking the muscles of the body and the brain, which lies within the protective cranium at the top of the spinal column.

We share this spinal column with our cousins, the great apes, which are also bipedal, albeit intermittently. As a result, our spinal column is different from theirs.

The spinal column: a stayed axis

The spinal column, the vertical axis of the body, must reconcile two contradictory mechanical requirements: rigidity and plasticity. It achieves this goal, despite the apparently unstable stacking of the vertebrae, as a result of **stays built into its very structure.**

In fact, when the body is in **the position of symmetry** (Fig. 1) the spinal column as a whole can be viewed as a ship's mast resting on the pelvis and extending to the head. At shoulder level it supports a main-yard set transversely (i.e. the shoulder girdle); at all levels it contains *ligamentous and muscular tighteners* arranged as **stays** linking the mast itself to its attachment site (i.e. the hull of the ship or the pelvis in the body).

A second system of stays is closely related to the scapular girdle and has the shape of a lozenge, with its long axis vertical and its short axis horizontal. When the body is in the position of symmetry, the tensions in the stays are balanced on both sides, and the mast is vertical and straight.

In **one-legged standing** (Fig. 2), when the body weight rests entirely on one lower limb, the pelvis tilts to the opposite side and the vertical column is forced to bend as follows:
- in the lumbar region it becomes convex towards the resting limb
- then concave in the thoracic region
- and finally convex once more in the cervical region.

The muscular tighteners *automatically* adapt their tension to restore equilibrium under the guidance of spinal reflexes and of the central nervous system, and this active adaptation is under the control of the extrapyramidal system, which constantly re-adjusts the tonus of the various postural muscles.

The plasticity of the spine resides in its make-up (i.e. multiple components superimposed on one another and interlinked by ligaments and muscles). Its shape can therefore be *altered by the muscular tighteners while its rigidity is maintained.* This is an example of biotensegrity.

Fig. 1

Fig. 2

The spinal column: axis of the body and protector of the neuraxis

The spinal column is in effect the **central pillar of the trunk** (Fig. 3). Its *thoracic segment* (cross-section **b**) lies more posteriorly, one-quarter deep in the thorax; its *cervical segment* (cross-section **a**) lies more centrally, one-third deep in the neck, and its *lumbar segment* (cross-section **c**) lies centrally in the middle of the trunk. Local factors can explain these variations in position as follows:

*   in the cervical region, the spine supports the head and must lie as close as possible below its centre of gravity
*   in the thoracic region, it is displaced posteriorly by the mediastinal organs, especially the heart
*   in the lumbar region, where it must support the weight of the entire upper trunk, it resumes a central position and juts into the abdominal cavity.

In addition to supporting the trunk, the spine is the **protector of the neuraxis** (Fig. 4): the vertebral canal starts at the foramen magnum and provides a flexible and efficient casing for the spinal cord. This protection, however, is not without its downside, since, under certain circumstances and at certain locations, the protective casing can come into conflict with the neuraxis and the spinal nerves, as we shall see later.

Figure 4 also shows the four segments of the spine:

*   the **lumbar segment** (1), where the lumbar vertebrae **L** are centrally located
*   the **thoracic segment** (2), where the vertebrae **T** lie posteriorly
*   the **cervical segment** (3), where the vertebrae **C** are almost central
*   the **sacrococcygeal segment** (4), formed by two composite bones **S**.

The **sacrum** is formed by the fusion of the five sacral vertebrae and is part of the pelvic girdle.

The **coccyx** articulates with the sacrum and is the vestige of the tail seen in most mammals. It is formed by the fusion of four to six tiny coccygeal vertebrae.

Below the *second lumbar vertebra* (L2), where lies the **conus medullaris**, the spinal canal contains only the **filum terminale internum**, which has no neurological function.

The site of mechanical weakness in the spinal column is at the level of the lumbosacral intervertebral disc (L5 -S1), which links the vertebrae of the sacrum and supports the entire weight of the upper part of the body and also any weights carried by the upper limbs, on the head or on the shoulders.

1/3   a

1/4   b

1/2   c

Fig. 3

3

C

T

2

1

L

S

4

Fig. 4

A global view of the spinal curvatures

The spine as a whole is straight when viewed **from the front or from the back** (Fig. 5). Some people may show a slight lateral curvature, which of course remains within normal limits.

In this position **the line of the shoulders** (s) and **the line of the sacral fossae** (p), which is the short diagonal of *Michaelis's lozenge* (red dotted line; see later, p. 82), are parallel and horizontal. On the other hand, **when viewed from the side** (i.e. in the sagittal plane; Fig. 6), the spine contains four curvatures, which are, caudocranially, the following:

- the **sacral curvature** (1), which is fixed as a result of the definitive fusion of the sacral vertebrae and is concave anteriorly
- the **lumbar curvature** or **lumbar lordosis** (2), which is concave posteriorly – when this concavity is exaggerated the term **lumbar hyperlordosis** is used
- the **thoracic curvature** (3), also called **thoracic kyphosis**, especially when it is accentuated

- the **cervical curvature** (4) or **cervical lordosis**, which is concave posteriorly and whose concavity is proportional to the degree of thoracic kyphosis.

In the well-balanced erect posture, the posterior part of the cranium, the back and the buttocks lie tangential to a vertical plane (e.g. a wall). The depth of each curvature is measured by the **perpendicular** drawn from this vertical plane to the apex of the curvature. These perpendiculars will be further defined later (see p. 119).

These curvatures offset each other so that the plane of the bite **b**, represented by a piece of cardboard held between the teeth, is horizontal and the eyes **h** are automatically directed **to the horizon.**

In the sagittal plane, these curvatures can be associated with *curvatures in the coronal plane*, known commonly as **humps** or medically as **scoliosis.**

Fig. 5

Fig. 6

The development of the spinal curvatures

During **phylogeny** (i.e. evolution from the **prehominids to Homo sapiens**) the transition from the quadruped to the biped state (Fig. 7) led first to the straightening and then to the *inversion of the lumbar curvature* (black arrows) from concave anteriorly to concave posteriorly (i.e. the lumbar lordosis).

In fact, the angle formed by the straightening of the trunk was only partially *absorbed* by retroversion of the pelvis, and bending of the lumbar column had to occur to absorb the rest. This explains the **lumbar lordosis**, which varies according to the degree of anteversion or retroversion of the pelvis. At the same time the cervical spine, which articulated with the cranium caudally, was progressively displaced anteriorly under the cranium so that the **foramen magnum moved forward towards the base of the skull** (arrow).

In *quadrupeds* the four limbs are weight-bearing (blue arrows), whereas in *bipeds* only the lower limbs are weight-bearing. Thus the lower limbs are now subject to *compression*, while the upper limbs, hanging free (red arrow), are subject to *elongation*.

During **ontogeny** (i.e. the development of the individual) similar changes can be seen in the lumbar region (Fig. 8, inspired by T.A. Willis). On the *first day of life* (a) the lumbar spine is concave anteriorly and at *5 months* (b) it is still slightly concave anteriorly. It is only at *13 months* (c) that the lumbar spine becomes straight. From *3 years* onwards (d) the lumbar lordosis begins to appear, becoming obvious by *8 years* (e) and assuming the definitive adult state at *10 years* (f).

Thus ontogeny recapitulates phylogeny.

Fig. 7

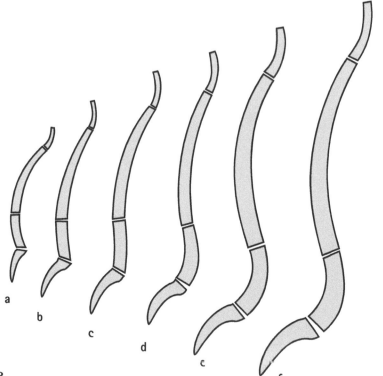

Fig. 8

Structure of the typical vertebra

Analysis of the structure of a typical vertebra reveals two major components:
- the vertebral body anteriorly
- the vertebral arch posteriorly.

A view of the typical vertebra disassembled (Fig. 9) reveals the following:
- the body (1), the larger cylindroid component, is wider than it is tall, with a cutoff corner posteriorly
- the posterior arch (2), U-shaped or horseshoe-shaped, receives on either side (Fig. 10) the articular processes (3 and 4), which divide the arch into two parts (Fig. 11):
    - the pedicles (8 and 9) in front of the articular processes
    - the laminae (10 and 11) behind the articular processes.

In the midline is attached the spinous process (7). The arch is then attached (Fig. 12) to the posterior surface of the body by the pedicles. The **complete vertebra** (Fig. 13) also contains the transverse processes (5 and 6), which are attached to the arch near the articular processes.

This typical vertebra is found *at all spinal levels* with, of course, profound alterations that affect either the body or the arch but generally both simultaneously.

It is important to note, however, that in *the vertical plane* all these various constituents are aligned in anatomical correspondence. As a result, the entire spine is made up of **three columns** (Fig. 14):
- one **major column** (A), anteriorly located and made up of the stacked vertebral bodies
- two **minor columns** (B and C), posterior to the body and made up of the stacked articular processes.

The bodies are joined to each other by intervertebral discs, and the articular processes to each other by plane synovial joints. Thus at the level of each vertebra there is a canal bounded by the body anteriorly and the arch posteriorly. These successive canals make up the **vertebral or spinal canal** (12), which is formed alternately by:
- bony structures at the level of each vertebra
- fibrous structures between the vertebrae (i.e. the intervertebral discs and the ligaments of the dorsal arch).

Fig. 9

Fig. 11

Fig. 10

Fig. 12

Fig. 13

Fig. 14

The legends are the same for all figures.

The spinal curvatures

The spinal curvatures **increase resistance** to axial compression forces. Engineers have shown (Fig. 15) that the resistance **R** of a curved column is directly proportional to the number **N** of curvatures plus 1 (with k being the proportionality factor). If a *straight column* (a) with N = 0 and R = 1 is taken as reference, then the column (b) with a single curvature has a resistance of 2 and a column with two curvatures (c) a resistance of 5. Finally, a column with *three flexible curvatures* (d), like the spine with its lumbar, thoracic and cervical curvatures, has a resistance of 10 (i.e. 10 times that of a straight column).

The significance of these curvatures can be quantitated by the **Delmas index** (Fig. 16), which can only be measured on the skeleton and is expressed as the ratio H/L × 100, where H is the height of the spinal column from the upper surface of S1 to the atlas, and L is its fully extended length from the upper surface of the sacrum to the atlas.

A spinal column with *normal curvatures* (a) has an index of 95% with normal limits of 94-96%. A spinal column with *exaggerated curvatures* (b) has a Delmas index of 94%, signifying a greater difference between the fully extended length of the column and its height. On the other hand, a spinal column with *attenuated curvatures* (c) (i.e. almost straight), has an index greater than 96%.

This anatomical classification is very important because it is related to the functional type of the spinal column. A. Delmas has in fact demonstrated that a column with pronounced curvatures (i.e. with an almost horizontal sacrum and a strong lumbar lordosis) is of the dynamic type, whereas a column with attenuated curvatures (i.e. with an almost vertical sacrum and a flat back) is of the static type.

$$R = k (N^2+1)$$

N = 0   R = 1

N = 1   R = 2

N = 2   R = 5

N = 3   R = 10

Fig. 15   a   b   c   d

Spinal index	low (< 94 %)	intermediate	high (> 96 %)
Spinal curvature	exaggerated	intermediate	attenuated
Spinal type	dynamic	intermediate	static

Delmas index ➡️ $\dfrac{H \text{ (height)} \times 100}{L \text{ (fully extended length)}}$

Fig. 16

Structure of the vertebral body

The vertebral body is **built like a short bone** (Fig. 17) (i.e. *egg-like*, with a dense bony *cortex* surrounding a *spongy medulla*). Its superior and inferior surfaces, called the **intervertebral or discal surfaces**, consist of thick cortical bone, which is thicker centrally where it is partly cartilaginous.

Its margin is rolled up into a **labrum** (L), which is derived from the epiphyseal disc and becomes fused to the rest of the discal surface (S) at 14-15 years of age. Abnormal ossification of this epiphyseal plate leads to vertebral epiphysitis or **Scheuermann's disease.**

A **verticofrontal section** of the vertebral body (Fig. 18) shows clearly the thick cortical bone lining its lateral surfaces, the superior and inferior cartilage-lined discal surfaces and the spongy centre of the body with bony trabeculae dispersed along the *lines of force*, which run as follows:

- *vertically*, between the superior and inferior surfaces
- *horizontally*, between the two lateral surfaces
- *obliquely*, between the inferior surface and the lateral borders.

A **sagittal section** (Fig. 19) shows these vertical trabeculae once more. In addition, there are two sheaves of *oblique fibres* in a **fan-like arrangement:**

- the first (Fig. 20), arising *from the superior surface*, runs through the two pedicles to reach the corresponding superior articular surfaces and the spinous process

- the second (Fig. 21), arising *from the inferior surface*, runs through the two pedicles to reach the corresponding inferior articular surfaces and the spinous process.

The crisscrossing of these three trabecular systems creates zones of strong resistance as well as one **zone of weaker resistance** – in particular, the triangle with its base lying on the anterior border of the vertebral body, and made up entirely of vertical trabeculae (Fig. 22).

This explains the occurrence of the **wedge-shaped compression fracture of the vertebra** (Fig. 23). An axial compressive force of 600 kg crushes the anterior part of the vertebral body, leading to a compression fracture, but a force of 800 kg is needed to crush the whole vertebra and make the posterior part collapse (Fig. 24). This type of fracture is the only one able to damage the spinal cord by encroaching on the spinal canal.

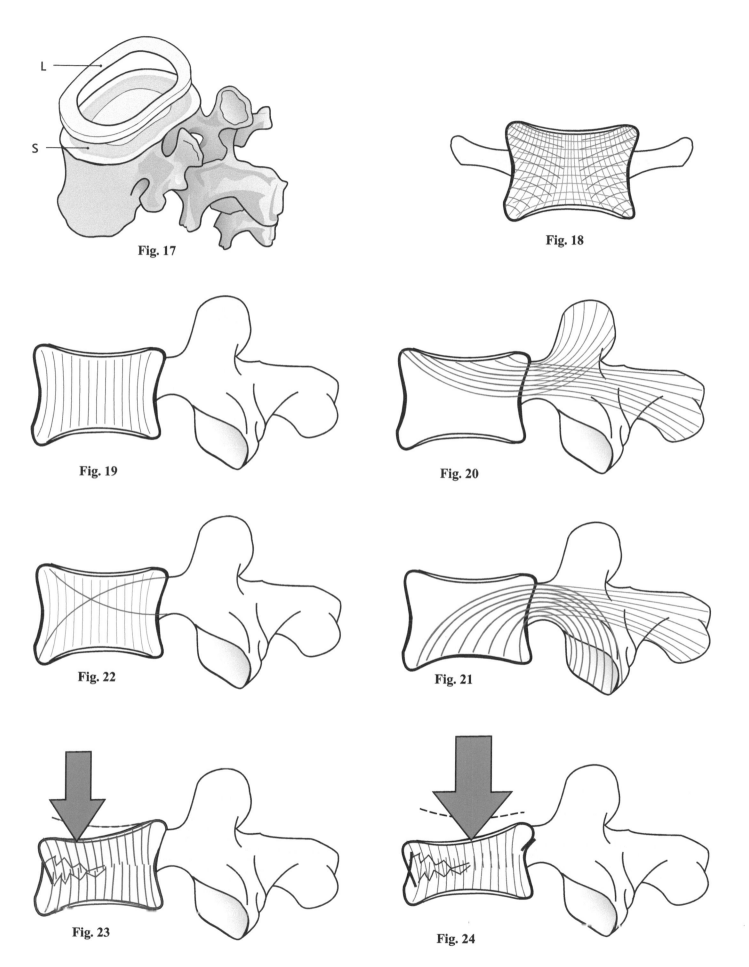

Fig. 17

Fig. 18

Fig. 19

Fig. 20

Fig. 22

Fig. 21

Fig. 23

Fig. 24

The functional components of a vertebra

When viewed laterally (Fig. 25, inspired by Brueger) the functional components of the vertebral column are easily distinguished:
- anteriorly (A) lies the vertebral body as part of the anterior pillar, which is essentially a supporting structure
- posteriorly (B) the posterior arch supports the articular processes, which are stacked together to form the posterior pillar.

While the anterior pillar plays a static role, the posterior pillar has a dynamic role to play.

In the **vertical plane** bony and ligamentous structures alternate, and give rise (according to Schmorl) to a **passive segment** (I) formed by the vertebra itself and a **mobile segment** (II), shown in blue in the diagram. The latter consists of the following:
- the intervertebral disc
- the intervertebral foramen
- the facet (zygapophyseal) joints (between the articular processes)
- the ligamentum flavum and the interspinous ligaments.

The mobility of this active segment is responsible for the movements of the vertebral spine.

There is a **functional link between the anterior and posterior pillars** (Fig. 26), formed by the pedicles. Each vertebra has a trabecular structure involving the body and the arch and can thus be likened to a lever of the first order, where the articular process (1) acts as the fulcrum. This first-class lever system, present at each vertebral arch, allows the axial compression forces acting on the column to be cushioned directly and passively (2) by the *intervertebral disc* and indirectly and actively by the paravertebral muscles (3). Thus the cushioning effect is **both passive and active.**

Fig. 25

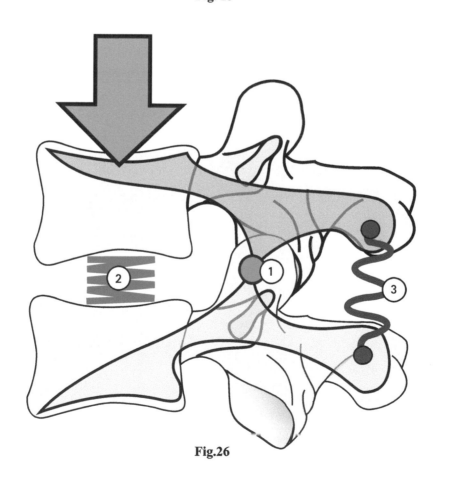

Fig.26

The elements of intervertebral linkage

Between the sacrum and the base of the skull there are **24 movable parts** (the vertebrae) linked together by many fibrous ligaments.

A horizontal section of a typical vertebra (Fig. 27) and a lateral view (Fig. 28) bring out the following ligaments:

- First, those attached to the **anterior pillar:**
  - the **anterior longitudinal ligament** (1), stretching from the cranial base to the sacrum on the anterior surfaces of the vertebral bodies
  - the **posterior longitudinal ligament** (2) extending from the jugular process of the occipital bone to the sacral canal on the posterior surfaces of the vertebral bodies.

These long ligaments are interlinked by each **intervertebral disc**, which consists peripherally of the **annulus fibrosus**, formed by concentric layers of fibrous tissue (6 and 7), and centrally of the **nucleus pulposus** (8).

- Second, the numerous ligaments **attached to the posterior arch** and connecting the arches of the adjacent vertebrae:
  - the strong thick **ligamentum flavum** (3), which meets its contralateral counterpart in the midline and is attached superiorly to the deep surface of the lamina of the upper vertebra and inferiorly to the superior margin of the lamina of the lower vertebra
  - the **interspinous ligament** (4), continuous posteriorly with the **supraspinous ligament** (5), which is poorly defined in the lumbar region but is quite distinct in the neck
  - the **intertransverse ligament** (10) attached to the apex of each transverse process
  - the two powerful **anterior and posterior ligaments** (9), which strengthen the capsules of the **facet joints.**

This ligamentous complex maintains an extremely solid link between the vertebrae and imparts a strong mechanical resistance to the spinal column. Only a severe trauma (e.g. a fall from a great height or a traffic accident) can cause rupture of these intervertebral linkages.

Fig. 27

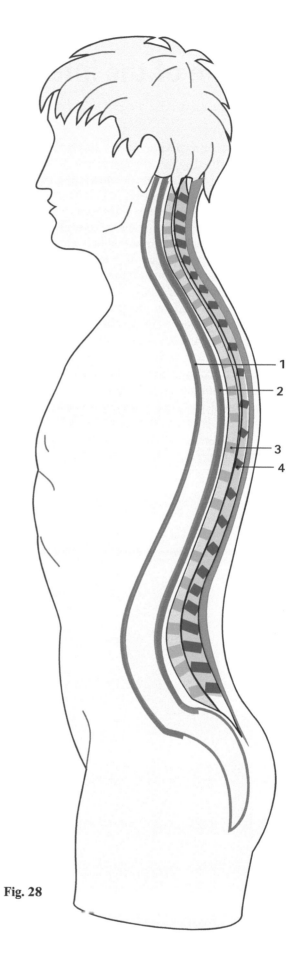

Fig. 28

Structure of the intervertebral disc

The joint between two vertebrae is a **symphysis** or **amphiarthrosis.** It is formed by the two adjacent vertebral discal surfaces and is connected by the **intervertebral disc**, whose structure is quite characteristic and consists of *two parts* (Fig. 29):

- A central part, the **nucleus pulposus** (N), a gelatinous substance derived embryologically from the *notochord*. It is a strongly hydrophilic transparent jelly containing 80% water; chemically it is made up of a *mucopolysaccharide* matrix containing protein-bound chondroitin sulphate, hyaluronic acid and keratan sulphate.

Histologically the nucleus comprises *collagenous fibres*, cells resembling *chondrocytes, connective tissue* cells and very few clusters of mature *cartilage* cells. **No blood vessels or nerves** penetrate the nucleus, and the absence of blood vessels excludes the possibility of spontaneous healing. It is hemmed in by fibrous tracts running from the margin.

- A peripheral part, the **annulus fibrosus** (A), made up of concentric fibres that *cross one another obliquely* in space from one layer to the next, as shown in the left half of the diagram (Fig. 30).

In the diagram on the right side (Fig. 31), the fibres are vertical peripherally and become *more oblique towards the centre*. The central fibres, in contrast to the nucleus pulposus, are nearly horizontal and run between the vertebral discal surfaces in an ellipsoid fashion. Thus the nucleus is enclosed within an *inextensible* casing between the two vertebral discal surfaces and the annulus, whose woven fibres prevent any extrusion of the nuclear substance in the young. The nucleus is **held under pressure** within its watertight casing so that when the disc is cut horizontally its gelatinous substance can be seen to bulge through the cut. This is also the case when the vertebral column is sectioned sagittally. This protrusion of the nucleus pulposus indicates that the gelatinous substance is under pressure.

Fig. 29

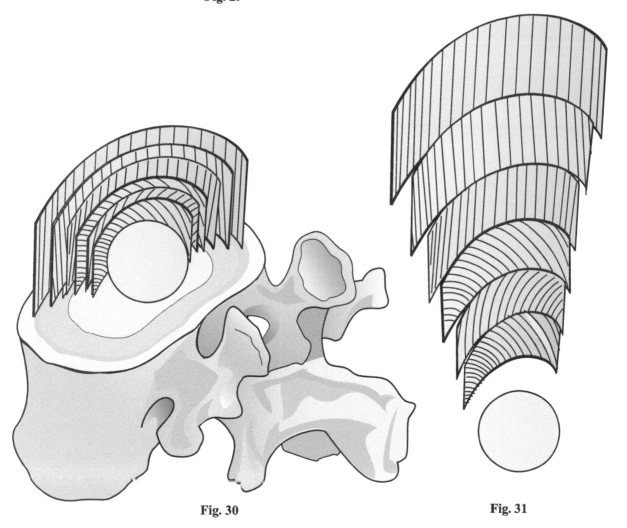

Fig. 30

Fig. 31

The nucleus pulposus likened to a swivel

Incarcerated under pressure within its casing between the two vertebral discal surfaces, the nucleus pulposus is **roughly spherical**. Therefore, as a first approximation, it can be compared to a billiard ball placed between two planes (Fig. 32). This type of joint, known in Mechanics as a swivel joint, allows three types of bending movement:

- in the sagittal plane, **flexion** (Fig. 33) or **extension** (Fig. 34)
- in the coronal plane, **lateral flexion**
- **rotation** of one discal surface relative to the other (Fig. 35).

In life the situation is more complex, since added to these movements occurring around the ball there are *gliding* and even *shearing* movements that take place between the two discal surfaces with the help of the ball. These movements take place while the nucleus rolls slightly in the direction of movement and is flattened on the side where the two discal surfaces are approximated.

During **flexion** (Fig. 36), the discal surface above is slightly displaced anteriorly, whereas in **extension** (Fig. 37) it is displaced posteriorly. Likewise, during **lateral flexion**, the displacement occurs on the side of bending. During **rotation** (Fig. 38) it takes place on the side of the rotation.

All told, this very mobile joint has exactly **six degrees of freedom:**

- flexion-extension
- lateral flexion on both sides
- gliding in the sagittal plane
- gliding in the transverse plane
- rotation to the right
- rotation to the left.

However, each of these movements has a small range, and sizable movements are only possible by the simultaneous participation of multiple joints.

These complex movements depend on the *arrangement of the posterior articular surfaces and of the ligaments*, which must be taken into account *in the design of disc prostheses* now under development.

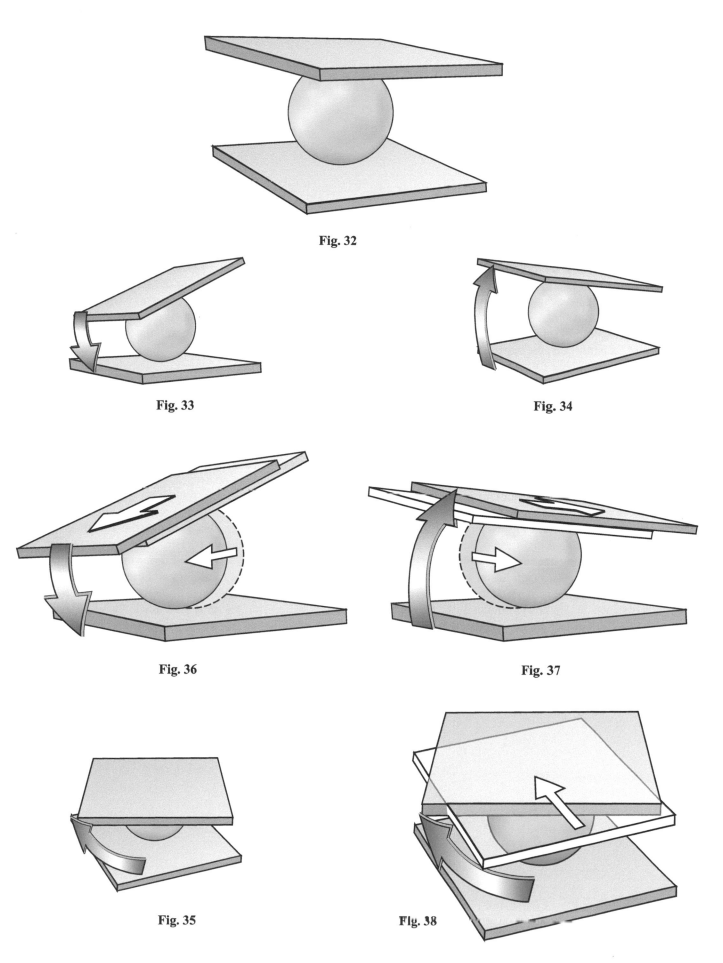

Fig. 32

Fig. 33

Fig. 34

Fig. 36

Fig. 37

Fig. 35

Fig. 38

The preloaded state of the disc and the self-stabilization of the disco-vertebral joint

The forces applied to the intervertebral disc are considerable, the more so as the sacrum is approached.

In terms of axial compression forces it has been worked out that when a vertebral discal surface presses on the disc **the nucleus pulposus bears 75% of the force and the annulus fibrosus bears the remaining 25%**, so that for a *force of 20 kg a 15-kg force is exerted on the nucleus and a 5-kg force on the annulus.*

In the horizontal plane, however, the nucleus **transmits** some of the pressure to the annulus (Fig. 39). For instance, in the standing position, the vertical compression force acting on the nucleus at L5-S1 level and transmitted to the margin of the annulus equals *28 kg/cm and 16kg/cm².* These forces are increased considerably when the subject is lifting a load. During forward flexion of the trunk the pressure/cm² rises to **58 kg**, while the force exerted/cm reaches **87 kg**. When the trunk is being brought back to the vertical, these pressures reach up to **107 kg/cm²** and **174 kg/cm**. These pressures can be higher still if a weight is lifted while the trunk is being straightened, and they come close to the values for breaking point.

The pressure in the centre of the nucleus is never zero, even when the disc is unloaded. This is due to the disc's water-absorbing capacity (hydrophilia), which *causes the disc to swell within its inextensible casing.* This is analogous to the **preloaded state**. In concrete-building technology preloading denotes a pre-existing tension within a beam about to be stressed. If a homogeneous beam (Fig. 40) is exposed to a load, it is deflected inwards for a distance denoted by f1 known as the *arrow*. These features of the preloaded state are now included in the new field of biotensegrity.

If a beam (Fig. 41) is fitted with a very taut cable passing through its lower half from one end (T) to the other (T'), it is now a preloaded beam*, and the deflexion f2 caused by the same load will be clearly smaller than f1.

The preloaded state of the disc likewise gives it greater resistance to the forces generated during axial compression and lateral flexion. As the nucleus loses its hydrophilic properties with age, its internal pressure decreases with **loss of its preloaded state**; hence the lack of *flexibility of the spinal column in the aged.*

When **an axial load is applied asymmetrically** to a disc (Fig. 42, F), the upper vertebral discal surface will tilt towards the overloaded side, making an angle (a) with the horizontal. Thus a fibre AB' will be stretched to AB but, at the same time, the internal pressure of the nucleus, which is maximal in the direction of the arrow (f), will act on that fibre AB and bring it back to AB', thereby righting the vertebral discal surface and restoring it to its original position. This **self-stabilization mechanism** is linked to the pre-loaded state. Therefore, the annulus and the nucleus form a **functional couple**, whose effectiveness depends on the integrity of each component. If the internal pressure of the nucleus decreases, or if the impermeability of the annulus is impaired, *this functional couple immediately loses its effectiveness.*

The preloaded state also explains the **elastic properties of the disc,** as well shown by Hirsch's experiment (Fig. 43). If a preloaded disc (P) is exposed to a **violent force** (S), the disc thickness exhibits a minimum and then a maximum, followed by *damped oscillations* over one second in accordance with the shock-absorption curve. If the force is too violent, the intensity of this oscillatory reaction can *destroy the fibres of the annulus,* accounting for the deterioration of intervertebral discs exposed to repeated violent stresses.

---

* The technique of using pre-stressed concrete, invented by the French engineer Eugene Freyssinet, has led to the construction of challenging buildings.

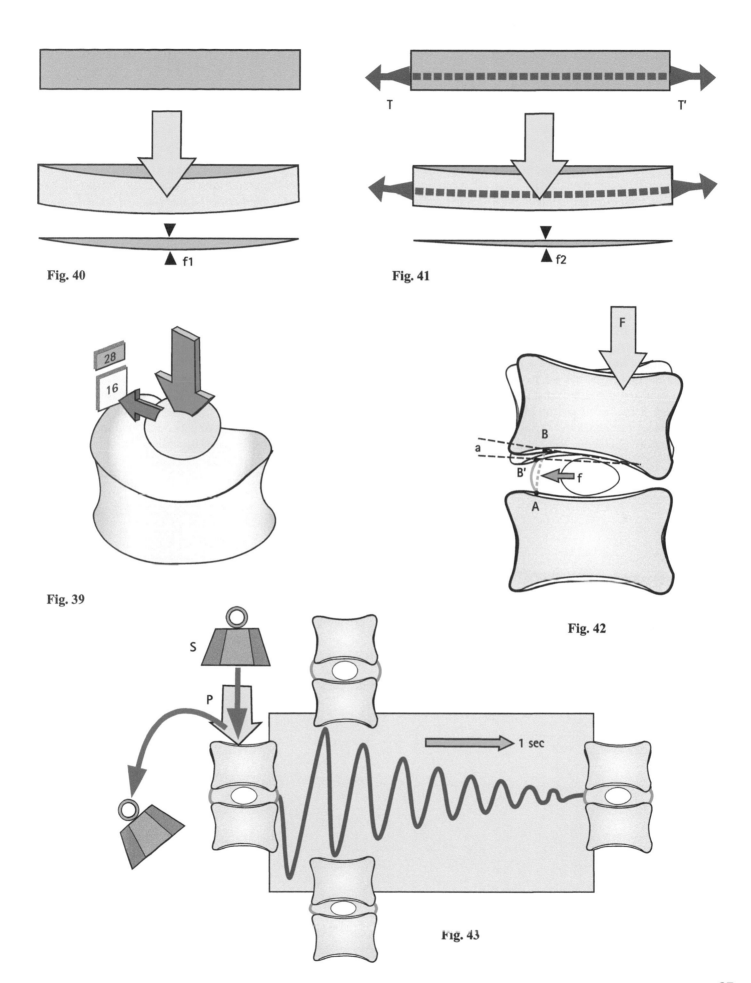

Fig. 40

Fig. 41

Fig. 39

Fig. 42

Fig. 43

27

Water imbibition by the nucleus pulposus

The nucleus rests on the centre of the vertebral discal surface, an area lined by cartilage and traversed by *many microscopic pores*, which link the casing of the nucleus with the spongy tissue underlying the vertebral discal surfaces. When a **significant axial force** is applied to the column, as by the weight of the body during standing (Fig. 44), the water contained in the gelatinous matrix of the nucleus escapes into the vertebral body through these pores (i.e. **the nucleus loses water**). As this static pressure is maintained throughout the day, by night *the nucleus contains less water than in the morning*, with the result that the disc is perceptibly thinner. In normal people this cumulative thinning of the discs during the day can amount to a loss in height of 2 cm. Conversely, *during the night*, in recumbency (Fig. 45), the vertebral bodies are no longer subject, to the axial force of gravity, but only to that generated by muscular tone, which is much reduced during sleep. In this **period of relief**, the hydrophilia of the nucleus draws water back into the nucleus from the vertebral body and the disc regains its original thickness (d). Therefore,

one is taller in the morning than at night. As the preloaded state is greater in the morning than at night, *the flexibility of the spinal column is greater in the morning.*

The imbibition pressure of the nucleus is considerable, since it can reach 250 mmHg (**Charnley**). With age, **its hydrated state is reduced** along with its hydrophilia and its state of preloading. This explains the *loss of height and of flexibility of the spinal column in the aged.*

As shown by **Hirsch**, when a constant load is applied to a vertebral disc (Fig. 46), the loss of thickness is *not linear but exponential* (first part of the curve), suggesting a dehydration process *proportional to the volume of the nucleus*. When the load is removed, the disc regains its initial thickness once more exponentially (second part of the curve), and the restoration to normal requires a finite time (T). If these forces are applied and removed over *too long a period*, the disc does not regain its initial length even if there is enough time for recovery. This results in **ageing of the vertebral disc.**

Fig. 44   **Fig. 45**

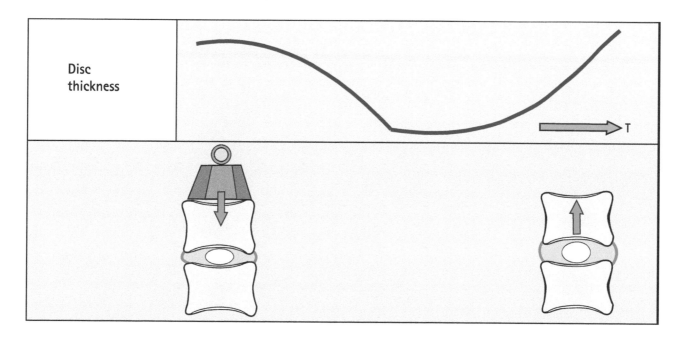

Disc
thickness

Fig. 46

Compressive forces acting on the disc

Compressive forces applied to the disc assume greater significance the nearer the disc is to the sacrum, because **the weight of the body supported** by the vertebral column increases with the length of the spinal column above (Fig. 47). For an 80-kg man the head weighs 3 kg, the upper limbs 14 kg and the trunk 30 kg. If it is assumed that at the level of disc L5-S1 the column supports only two-thirds of the weight of the trunk, then the weight borne is 37 kg, i.e. nearly half of the *body weight* **P**. To this must be added the *force exerted tonically by the paraspinal muscles* (M1 and M2) in order to maintain the trunk in the erect position at rest. If a *load* **E** is being carried and a further load **F** is added violently, the lowest discs may be subjected to forces that occasionally exceed their resistance, especially in the aged. The loss of thickness of the disc varies according to whether it is healthy or diseased. If a healthy disc at rest (Fig. 48) is loaded with a 100-kg weight, it is flattened by a distance of **1.4 mm** and becomes wider (Fig. 49). If a diseased disc is similarly loaded, it is flattened by a distance of **2 mm** (Fig. 50), and it fails to *recover completely its initial thickness* after unloading.

This progressive flattening of the disc is not without an effect on the facet joints:

* *with normal disc thickness* (Fig. 51) the cartilaginous articular facets of these joints are normally arranged, and their interspaces are straight and regular
* *with a flattened disc* (Fig. 52) the relationships of these facets are disturbed, and generally speaking the interspaces open out posteriorly.

This articular distortion, in the long run, is the main factor leading to **spinal osteoarthritis.**

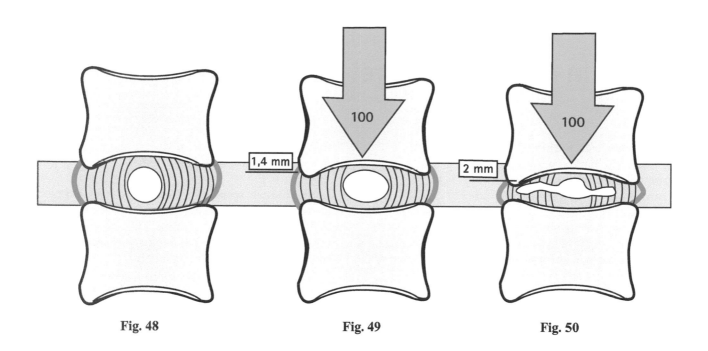

| Fig. 48 | Fig. 49 | Fig. 50 |

Fig. 47

Fig. 51

Fig. 52

Variations in disc structure related to cord level

Disc thickness varies with position in the spinal column:
- it is thickest in the lumbar region (Fig. 55), i.e. **9 mm**
- it is **5 mm** thick in the thoracic region (Fig. 54)
- it is **3 mm** thick in the cervical region (Fig. 53) i.e., the minimal thickness.

But more important than its absolute thickness is the **ratio** of disc thickness to the height of the vertebral body. In fact it is this ratio that accounts for the mobility of a particular segment of the column, since *the greater the ratio, the greater the mobility.* Thus, in decreasing order:
- the cervical spine (Figs 53 and 56) is the most mobile with a disc/body ratio of 2/5
- the lumbar spine (Figs 55 and 58) is slightly less mobile with a ratio of 1/3
- the thoracic spine (Figs 54 and 57) is the least mobile with a ratio of 1/5.

Sagittal sections of the various segments of the spine show that the nucleus pulposus is not exactly at the centre of the disc. If the antero-posterior thickness of the disc is divided into 10 equal parts, then:
- **In the cervical spine** (Fig. 56) the nucleus lies at 4/10ths thickness from the anterior border and 3/10ths thickness from the posterior border of the vertebra and occupies the intermediate 3/10ths. It *lies exactly on the axis of movement* (blue arrow).
- **In the thoracic spine** (Fig. 57) the nucleus is a little closer to the anterior than the posterior border. Once more it amounts to 3/10ths of the disc thickness, but it now lies posterior to the axis of movement. The blue arrow indicating this axis runs clearly anterior to the nucleus.
- **In the lumbar spine** (Fig. 58) the nucleus lies clearly closer to the posterior border, i.e. at 2/10ths thickness from the posterior border and 4/10ths thickness from the anterior border, but it now amounts to 4/10ths of the thickness, i.e. it has a greater surface area corresponding to the greater axial forces exerted there. As in the cervical spine it lies exactly on the axis of movement (blue arrow).

Leonardi considers that the centre of the nucleus **is equidistant from the anterior border of the vertebra and the ligamentum flavum** and corresponds obviously to a point of equilibrium, as if the strong posterior ligaments *acted to pull* the nucleus posteriorly.

Fig. 53

Fig. 54

Fig. 55

Fig. 56

Fig. 57

Fig. 58

Elementary movements in the intervertebral disc

Let us start with movements occurring in the axis of the spinal column. In the **rest position** (Fig. 59) before any loading, the fibres of the annulus fibrosus (3), already stretched by the nucleus pulposus (2), are in the **preloaded state.**

- When the **column is actively elongated** axially (Fig. 60, red arrows) the vertebral discal surfaces (1) tend to move apart, thus increasing the disc thickness (d). At the same time, its *width is reduced* and the tension in the annulus rises. The nucleus, somewhat flattened at rest, now becomes more spherical. This increase in disc height reduces the internal pressure; hence the rationale underlying *the treatment of disc prolapse by spinal traction*. When the spine is elongated, the gelatinous substance of the prolapsed disc moves back into its original intranuclear location. This result, however, is not always achieved, because the tightening of the central fibres of the annulus may in fact raise the internal pressure of the nucleus.

- **During axial compression** (Fig. 61, blue arrows), *the disc is crushed and widened and the nucleus is flattened so that its raised internal pressure* is transmitted laterally to the innermost fibres of the annulus. Thus a vertical force is transformed into lateral forces and stretches the fibres of the annulus.

- **During extension** (Fig. 62, red arrow) the upper vertebra moves posteriorly (p), reducing the intervertebral space and driving the nucleus anteriorly (blue arrow). The nucleus then presses on the anterior fibres of the annulus and increases their tension, with the result that the *upper vertebra is restored to its original position.*

- **During flexion** (Fig. 63, blue arrow) the upper vertebra moves anteriorly, narrowing the intervertebral space anteriorly (a). The nucleus is displaced posteriorly and now presses on the posterior fibres of the annulus, increasing their tension. Once more **self-stabilization** is the result of *the con-certed action of the nucleus-annulus couple in accordance with biotensegrity.*

- **During lateral flexion** (Fig. 64) the upper vertebra tilts towards the side of flexion and the nucleus is driven to the opposite side (green arrow). This results again in self-stabilization.

- **During axial rotation** (Fig. 65, blue arrows) the oblique fibres, running counter to the direction of movement, are stretched, while the intermediate fibres with opposite orientation are relaxed. The tension is maximal in the central fibres of the annulus, which are the most oblique. The nucleus is therefore *strongly compressed* and its internal pressure *rises in proportion to the degree of rotation*. This explains why combined flexion and axial rotation will tend to *tear the annulus* by increasing the pressure inside the nucleus and *driving it posteriorly* through potential cracks in the annulus.

- When a **static force is applied slightly obliquely to a vertebra** (Fig. 66), the vertical force (white arrow) can be resolved into:
  - a **force perpendicular** to the lower vertebral discal surface (blue arrow)
  - a **force parallel** to the same discal surface (red arrow).

The vertical force presses the two vertebrae together; the tangential force makes the upper vertebra slide anteriorly, and leads to progressive stretching of the oblique fibres in each fibrous layer of the annulus.

On the whole it is clear that, whatever the force applied to the disc, it **always increases the internal pressure of the nucleus and stretches the fibres of the annulus.** But, because of the relative movement of the nucleus, stretching the annulus fibrosus tends to oppose this movement; hence the system tends to be restored to its initial state.

Fig. 60

Fig. 59

Fig. 61

Fig. 62

Fig. 63

Fig. 64

Fig. 65

Fig. 66

Automatic rotation of the spine during lateral flexion

During lateral flexion the vertebral bodies automatically rotate on each other so that the line passing through the middle of their anterior surfaces is displaced contralaterally. This is clearly seen in the schematic representation of an **anterior radiograph taken during lateral flexion** (Fig. 67). The bodies lose their symmetry and the interspinous line (heavy broken line) moves towards the side of movement. One vertebra is drawn with its bony constituents to allow a better understanding of its orientation and of the radio-graphic findings.

When viewed from above (Fig. 68A), as the vertebra rotates, the transverse process on the side of lateral flexion appears in full view, whereas the contralateral process is foreshortened. Furthermore, the X-ray beam goes successively through the *facet joints* on the convex side (Fig. 68B), while providing a frontal view of these joints and of the vertebral pedicle on the concave side.

This automatic rotation of the vertebral bodies depends on two mechanisms:

- compression of the intervertebral discs
- stretching of the ligaments.

The effect of disc compression is easily displayed using a simple **mechanical model** (Fig. 69), which you can build as follows:

- Use wedge-shaped segments of cork and soft rubber to represent the vertebrae and the disc respectively.
- Glue them together.
- Draw a line centrally on their anterior surfaces to indicate the symmetrical resting position.
- Then bend the model laterally, and you will observe contralateral rotation of the vertebral bodies, indicated by the displacement of the various segments of the central line running through the vertebrae. Lateral bending increases the internal pressure of the disc on the concave side; as the disc itself is wedge-shaped, its compressed contents tend to

escape towards the more open side, i.e. the convex side. This leads to rotation.

This pressure differential is shown in Figure 68A, where a plus sign inside a circle marks the high pressure area and the arrow indicates the direction of rotation.

Conversely, lateral bending stretches the contralateral ligaments, which tend to move towards the midline so as to minimize their lengths. This is shown in Figure 68A as a circled minus sign at the level of an intertransverse ligament, while the arrow indicates the direction of movement.

It is remarkable that these two mechanisms are synergistic and contribute to rotation of the vertebrae *in the same direction*. This rotation is *physiological* but, in certain cases, the **vertebrae are fixed in a position of rotation**, as a result of an imbalance of the ligaments or of developmental abnormalities. This results in scoliosis, which combines fixed lateral flexion of the spine with rotation of the vertebral bodies.

This abnormal rotation can be demonstrated clinically as follows:

- in the normal subject (Fig. 70), when the trunk is flexed forwards, the spinal column is symmetrical posteriorly
- in the scoliotic subject (Fig. 71), when the trunk is flexed forwards, the column becomes *asymmetrical*, with the appearance of **a hump in the thoracic region** on *the same side as the convexity*. The diagnosis of scoliosis is initially made clinically.

This is the result of a state of *permanent rotation of the vertebrae*. Thus in **scoliosis** the short-lasting physiological automatic rotation of the vertebral bodies has become pathological in being permanently linked to spinal flexion. Since it occurs in the young, this deformity becomes fixed as a result of unequal growth of the vertebral bodies.

Fig. 67

Fig. 68

Fig. 69

Fig. 70

Fig. 71

Global ranges of movement during flexion-extension of the spine

Taken as a whole, the column from **sacrum to skull** corresponds to a **joint with three degrees of freedom** allowing the following movements:

- flexion-extension
- lateral flexion to the right and to the left
- axial rotation.

It is thus **equivalent to a ball-and-socket joint** placed **between the sacrum and the skull**.

The ranges of these various elementary movements at each level of the spine are quite small, but their cumulative effect is significant in view of the many joints involved (i.e. **25 in all**, discounting the sacrococcygeal joint).

Flexion-extension takes place in the sagittal plane (Fig. 72). The reference plane at skull level is the **plane of the bite**, which can be imagined as a sheet of cardboard tightly held between the teeth. The angle formed by the plane of the bite and the two extreme positions **Tr** is 250° in the normal subject. To measure this angle the direction of the arrow that represents the plane of the bite must be taken into account. This range is considerable when compared to the 180° maximum range of all the other joints of the body. Of course this 250° value applies to the maximum range attained in normal supple individuals. The young can do a crab (Fig. 73), but at all ages it is easier to curl up in flexion (Fig. 74). On the other hand, these ranges can be even greater in certain male or female acrobats who can push their heads between their thighs (see Fig. 19, page 321).

The segmental contributions can be measured on **lateral** radiographs:

- **in the lumbar spine, flexion** (blue arrow) attains 60° and **extension** (red arrow) 20°
- **for the thoracolumbar spine** taken as a whole: **flexion** attains 60° and **extension** 60°
- **for the thoracic spine** the ranges can be calculated by subtraction, i.e. flexion (Fts) = 45° and extension (Ets) = 40°
- **for the cervical spine** (Fig. 75) the range of movement is measured between the upper discal surface of the first thoracic vertebra and the plane of the bite. It attains **60° for extension** and **40° for flexion**, giving a total range of close to 100°.

For **the total range of movement of the spine** the double black arrows indicate the axes of reference.

The **total range of flexion of the spine** (Ft) is thus 110° and **total extension** (Et) is 140°. When added together, the total range (Tr) is 250°, which greatly exceeds the 180° limit of all the other joints.

Nonetheless these figures are given as guidelines, as there is no agreement among authors regarding the range of movement at the various levels of the spine. Moreover, these values vary enormously with age. Therefore only **maximum values** for non-acrobats are given here.

Et = 140°

60°
Ets = 40°

Ft = 110°

105°
Fts = 45°

60°

20°

Tr = 250°

Fig. 72

60°

40°

Fig. 75

Fig. 73

Fig. 74

Global ranges of lateral flexion of the spine

Lateral flexion occurs in a coronal plane (Fig. 76). Clinically these ranges cannot be measured accurately, but it is easy to measure them on **radiographs taken from the front** (Fig. 77) using as reference either the axis of the vertebrae or the orientation of the upper surface of a particular vertebra. The baseline is the **lumbosacral articular surface**, i.e. the upper surface of the first sacral vertebra.

At skull level the landmark is the **intermastoid line**, i.e. the line passing through the two mastoid processes.
- Lateral flexion of the **lumbar spine** (L) attains 20°.
- Lateral flexion of the **thoracic spine** (TH) attains 20°.
- Lateral flexion of the **cervical spine** (C) is 35-45°.
- The total range of flexion of the spine (T) from sacrum to cranium is 75-85° on each side.

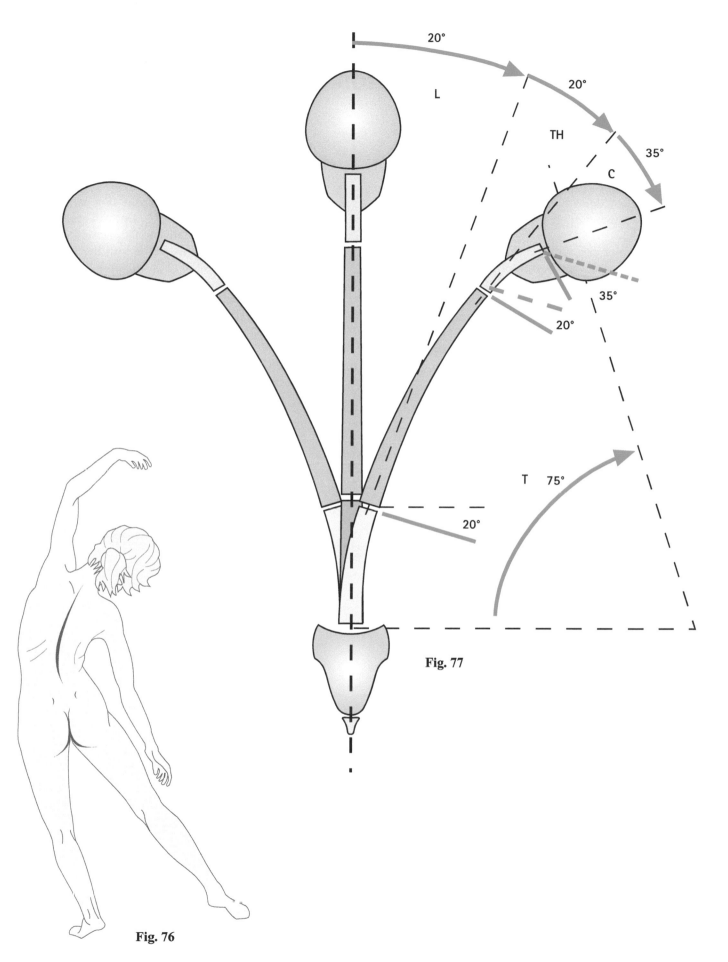

Fig. 76

Fig. 77

20°

20°

L

TH

35°

C

35°

20°

20°

T 75°

Global ranges of axial rotation of the spine

It is difficult to measure the ranges of axial rotation clinically. Moreover, it is impossible to take radiographs in the transverse planes, and axial CT scans need to be taken to measure this rotation precisely. Clinically the total rotation of the spine can be measured by fixing the pelvis and noting the angle of rotation of the skull.

Recently, two American authors (Gregersen and Lucas) have been able to measure very accurately the elementary components of rotation by using metal chips inserted into the spinous processes under local anaesthesia. We will come back to this work later when dealing with the thoracolumbar spine.

- Axial rotation of the **lumbar spine** (Fig. 78) is quite small, only 5°. The reasons for this will become apparent later.

- Axial rotation of the **thoracic spine** (Fig. 79) is more extensive, i.e. 35°. It is enhanced by the arrangement of the articular processes.

- Axial rotation of the **cervical spine** (Fig. 80) is definitely more extensive, attaining 45-50°. One can see that the atlas has rotated almost 90° relative to the sacrum.

- Axial rotation between **the pelvis and the skull** (Fig. 81) attains or just exceeds 90°. The *atlanto-occipital joint contributes a few degrees of rotation* but, as very often the range of rotation in the thoracolumbar region is smaller than expected, total rotation barely attains 90°.

Fig. 78

Fig. 79

Fig. 80

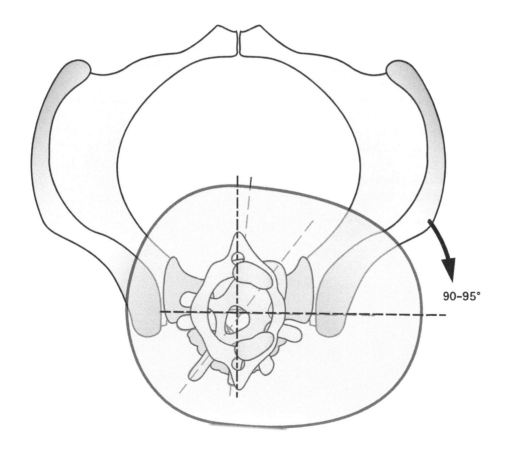

Fig. 81

Clinical assessment of the global ranges of spinal movements

Accurate measurements of the global ranges of spinal movements can only be made using radiographs of the entire column for flexion-extension and lateral flexion, and CT scans for rotation. Nevertheless these ranges can be obtained clinically with the use of certain 'test' measurements:

- **For flexion of the thoracolumbar spine** (Fig. 82) proceed as follows:
  - Measure the angle **a** between the vertical line **V** and the line joining the anterosuperior border of the greater trochanter to the lateral extremity of the acromion. This angle also includes a contribution of flexion at the hip.
  - Or determine the **level attained by the tips of the fingers** (f) during flexion of the trunk in the standing position with knees extended; here again some hip flexion is included. Then measure in centimetres the distance **f** from the fingertips to the ground or the distance **n** from the level of the fingertips to a landmark in the lower limbs, e.g. patella, mid-calf, instep or toes.
  - Or measure quite roughly with a tape the distance between the spinous processes of C7 and S1 during extension and flexion. In the diagram this distance increases by 5 cm in flexion.
- **For extension of the thoracolumbar spine** (Fig. 83) proceed as follows:
  - Measure the angle **a** between the vertical line **V** and the line joining the anterosuperior border of the greater trochanter to the lateral extremity of the acromion during maximal extension. This value also includes some degree of extension at the hips.
  - Or (to be slightly more accurate) measure the angle of extension of the spine in its entirety (angle **b**) and then

subtract from it the angle of extension of the cervical column (measured by keeping the trunk vertical and throwing the head backwards). A good test of extension and flexibility of the column is to 'do the crab' (see Fig. 73, p. 39), but its usefulness is clearly limited.

- **For lateral flexion of the thoracolumbar spine** (Fig. 84), proceed as follows:
  - Measure from behind the angle **a** between the vertical line **V** and the line joining the upper edge of the natal cleft to the spinous process of C7. It would be more accurate, however, to measure the angle **b** between the vertical line and the tangent to the curvature of the spine at C7. A simpler and quicker method is to determine the level **n** of the fingertips with respect to the position of the knee on the side of bending (i.e. where it lies above or below the knee).
- **For axial rotation** (Fig. 85):
  - Examine from above the subject, who sits on a low-backed chair with the pelvis fixed by steadying both pelvis and knees. The plane of reference is the coronal plane **C** passing across the top of the head, and the rotation of the thoracolumbar spine is measured by the angle **a** between the shoulder line **Sh–Sh′** and the coronal plane.
- **For the range of rotation of the entire spinal column:**
  - measure the angle of rotation **b** between the interauricular line and the coronal plane
  - or measure the angle of rotation **b′** between the plane of symmetry of the head **S′** and the sagittal plane **S**.

Fig. 82

Fig. 83

Fig. 84

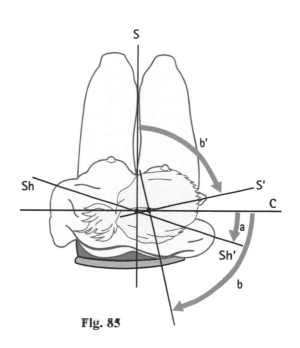

Fig. 85

Chapter 2

THE PELVIC GIRDLE

The pelvic girdle, also called the **pelvis**, is the base of the trunk and the very **foundation of the abdomen.** It also **links** the lower limbs to the vertebral column and, as a result, it **supports the entire body.**

With respect to its prototype in the vertebrates it is an anatomical structure that has undergone **extensive changes**, particularly in mammals and later in the great apes and in Homo sapiens. The pelvic cavity contains not only some abdominal organs but also, in women, the uterus, which grows considerably during pregnancy. As a result, the **perineum** (i.e. the pelvic diaphragm) has been shaped to allow the expulsion of the fetus by the mechanism of **labour.**

The pelvic girdle in the two sexes

The pelvic girdle is made up of three bony parts:
- the two iliac bones, paired and symmetrical
- the sacrum, unpaired but symmetrical, a solid piece of bone resulting from the fusion of five sacral vertebrae.

It has three joints with limited movements:
- the two sacroiliac joints between the sacrum and each iliac bone
- the pubic symphysis linking the iliac bones anteriorly.

Taken as a whole, the pelvic girdle resembles a funnel with its broader base facing superiorly and forming the pelvic inlet, which links the abdominal and pelvic cavities.

Sexual dimorphism, i.e. the structural differences in the two sexes, is obvious in the pelvic girdle:
- When the male pelvis (Fig. 1) and the female pelvis (Fig. 2) are compared, the latter is found to be much *wider* and much more *flared*. Thus the triangle enclosing the female pelvis has a much wider base than that enclosing the male pelvis.
- On the other hand, the female pelvis is much shorter than the male pelvis so that the trapezium enclosing it is lower.
- Finally, the pelvic inlet (unbroken black line) is proportionately much longer and more wide-mouthed in the female.

This structural difference in the pelvic girdle is related to **gestation**, and especially **labour**, since the fetus, particularly its relatively large head, *lies initially above the pelvic inlet*, which it must cross *before entering the cavity* and *exiting via the pelvic outlet*.

The joints of the pelvic girdle therefore are not only important in **determining the static properties of the erect trunk at rest and during walking** but also **participate actively in the mechanism of labour**, as we shall see in our discussion of the sacroiliac joint and the pubic symphysis.

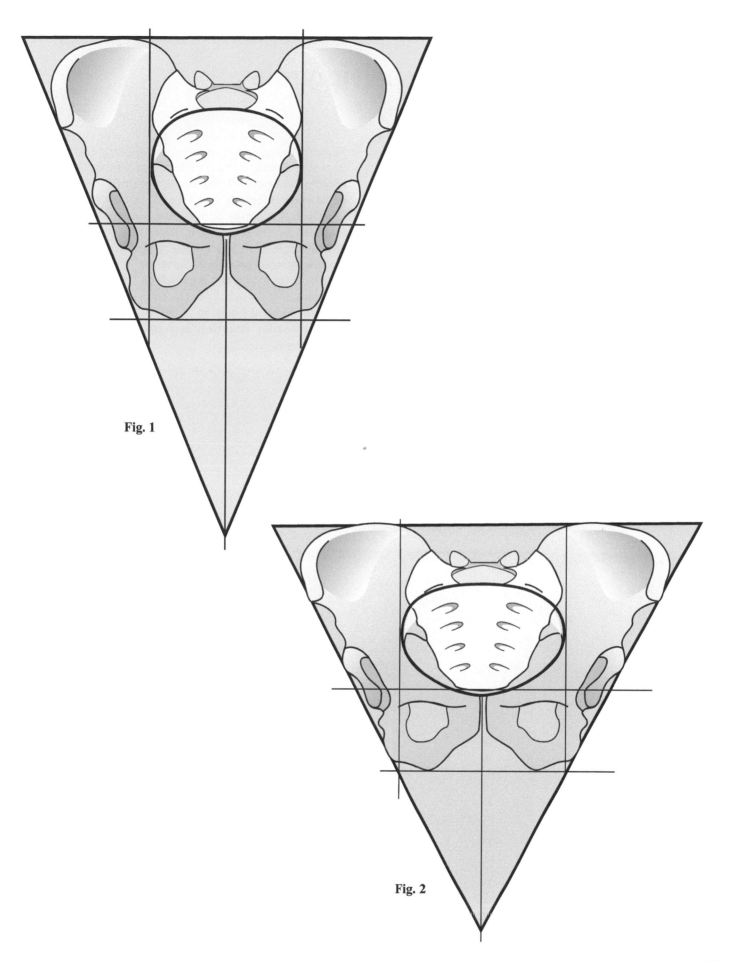

Fig. 1

Fig. 2

49

Mechanical model of the pelvic girdle

Mechanically speaking the pelvic girdle (Fig. 3) consists of three bony parts:

- the sacrum
- the two iliac bones.

The symmetrical, wedge-shaped **sacrum**, which lies in the midline, forms the base of the spine and fits like a keystone between the **iliac bones**, which are joined anteriorly at the pubic symphysis.

Each iliac bone (Fig. 4), which articulates with the sacrum, consists of **two roughly flat parts**, (i.e. the **ilium** above and the **fused pubis** and **ischium** enclosing the obturator foramen below). These parts form an **angle** with each other such that the whole bone recalls the two planes formed by the blades of a **propeller.**

These two parts fuse in the **acetabulum** (Fig. 5), which corresponds to the **axis of the propeller** and forms the **hip joint** with the femoral head.

These two roughly flat parts form a solid angle opening inwards (Fig. 6) and provide sites of attachment for the powerful muscles of the pelvic girdle. Their two upper surfaces make an **obtuse angle open anteriorly** (Fig. 3) and combine with the spine posteriorly and centrally to form the posterior wall of the lower abdomen, i.e. the **false pelvis.** Their two lower surfaces make an **obtuse angle open posteriorly**, and combine with the sacrum posteriorly and centrally to form the inferior compartment of the pelvic cavity, i.e. the **true pelvis.** The pelvic girdle has two functions:

- a **mechanical function** as part of the skeleton of the trunk
- a **protective function** in supporting and containing the abdominal viscera.

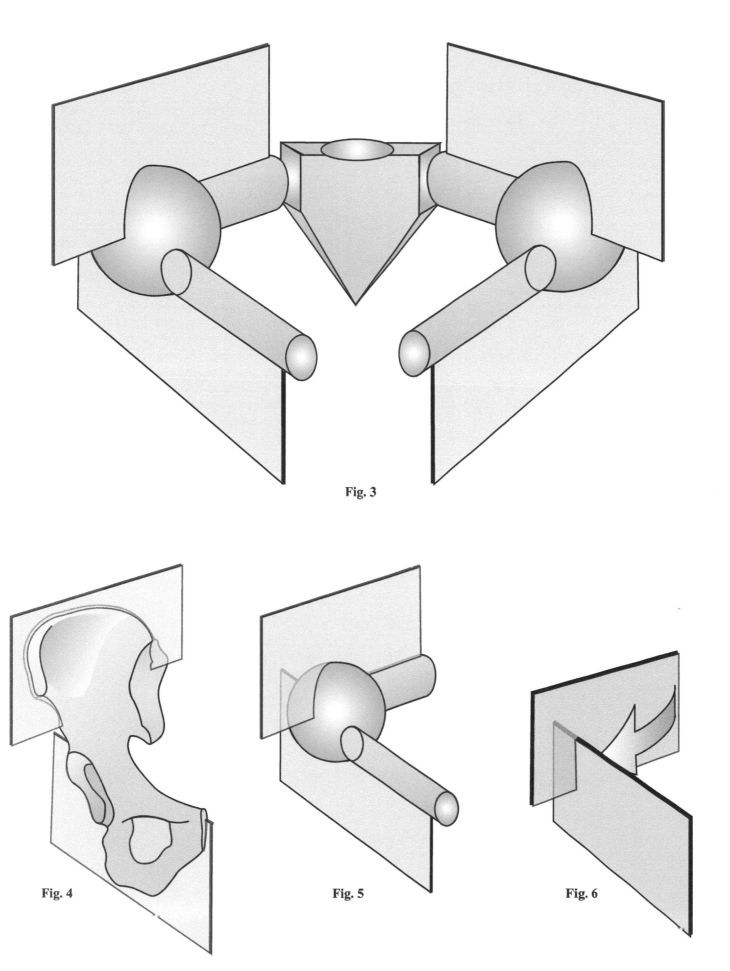

Fig. 3

Fig. 4

Fig. 5

Fig. 6

51

Architecture of the pelvic girdle

The pelvic girdle transmits forces between the spine and the lower limbs (Fig. 7). The weight (P), supported by L5, is distributed equally along the **alae of the sacrum** and through the ischial tuberosities towards the **acetabulum.**

The resistance of the ground (R) to the body weight is transferred to the acetabulum by the neck and head of the femur. Part of this resistance is transmitted across the **horizontal ramus of the pubic bone** and counterbalanced at the pubic symphysis by a similar force from the opposite side.

These lines of force form a complete ring acting along the **pelvic inlet.** There is a complex system of bony trabeculae to direct these forces through the bony pelvis (see Volume 2). As the wide sacrum is broader above than below, it can be considered a wedge (triangle) embedded vertically between the iliac bones. It is **suspended from these bones by ligaments**, and as a result it is more tightly held the heavier the weight it is carrying. It is thus a **self-locking system.**

The sacrum also fits between the iliac bones in the transverse plane (Figs 8 and 9). Each iliac bone can be viewed as the **arm of a lever** (Fig. 8) with its fulcrum (O1 and O2) located at the **sacroiliac joint** and its resistance force and its effort force acting on their anterior and posterior extremities, respectively. Posteriorly the resistance force would reside in the powerful **sacroiliac ligaments** (L1 and L2) and anteriorly the effort force would act at the pubic symphysis subjected to two approximately equal forces (S1 and S2).

When the **symphysis is dislocated** (Fig. 9) the separation (**diastasis**) of the two pubic bones (S) causes the iliac bones to move apart at the sacroiliac joints and thus frees up the sacrum, which can now move forwards (d1 and d2).

Whenever the lower limb presses on the ground the dislocated pelvic ring undergoes a shearing motion at the symphysis (Fig. 10). Thus any local break in the ring affects it as a whole and decreases its mechanical resistance.

Fig. 7

Fig. 8

Fig. 9

Fig. 10

The articular surfaces of the sacroiliac joint

When a sacroiliac joint (Fig. 11, right side) is opened like a book by swivelling its bony components about a vertical axis (line of dots and dashes), the auricular surfaces are clearly seen to match each other.

- The **auricular surface of the iliac bone** (A) lies on the posterosuperior part of the internal aspect of the bone just posterior to the iliopectineal line, which forms part of the pelvic inlet. It is crescent-shaped, concave posterosuperiorly and lined by cartilage. As a whole the surface is quite irregular, but Farabeuf claims that it has the shape of a *segment of rail*. In fact, its long axis contains a long crest lying between two furrows. This curved crest corresponds roughly to an arc of a circle whose centre lies approximately at the **sacral tuberosity** (black cross). As we shall see later, this tuberosity is the site of attachment of the **powerful sacroiliac ligaments.**
- The **auricular surface of the sacrum** (B) corresponds in shape and surface contours to that of the iliac bone. In its centre there is a curved **furrow** bordered by two long crests and corresponding to an arc of a circle whose centre lies on the transverse tubercle of S1 (black cross), where the powerful sacroiliac ligaments are attached. Farabeuf claims that this auricular surface has the shape of a *tramrail*, corresponding exactly to the rail-like surface of the iliac bone. These two surfaces, however, are not as regular as described above, and the three horizontal sections of the sacroiliac joint show that only in its superior (Fig. 12) and middle (Fig. 13) portions does the auricular facet of the sacrum contain a central furrow, while its inferior (Fig. 14) portion is more or less convex. As a result, it is very difficult to run a single X-ray beam along the sacroiliac joint, and therefore the beam will need to be fired obliquely lateromedially or mediolaterally, depending on the part under study.

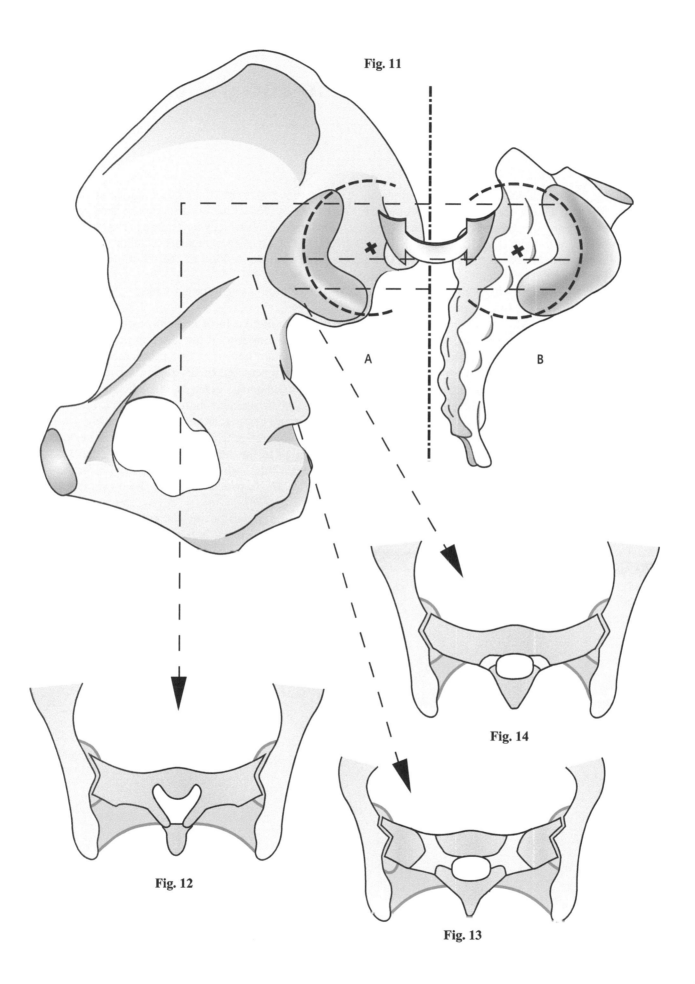

Fig. 11

Fig. 12

Fig. 13

Fig. 14

A

B

The auricular facet of the sacrum and the various spinal types

The **sacral auricular facet** is subject to wide structural variations from person to person, and A. Delmas has demonstrated a correlation between the spinal functional type and the shape of the sacrum and of its auricular facet (Fig. 15).
- **When the spinal curvatures are very pronounced** (A), i.e. the **dynamic type**, the *sacrum lies quite horizontally* and *its auricular facet is at once bent on itself* and quite deep. The sacroiliac joint is **highly mobile** like a typical synovial joint and represents *a state of overadaptation to bipedalism.*
- **When the curvatures of the column are poorly developed** (C), i.e. the **static type**, the sacrum is almost vertical, and its auricular facet is very elongated vertically, **minimally buckled on itself** and almost flat. This auricular facet has a very different shape from that described by Farabeuf and corresponds to a **joint of low mobility** like a symphysis. It is often seen in children and closely resembles that found in primates.
- There is also an **intermediate type** (B) lying between these two extremes.

A. Delmas has shown that **during evolution from primates to humans**, the caudal segment of the auricular facet becomes longer and wider and assumes in humans greater significance than the cranial segment. The angle between these two segments can reach 90° in humans, while in primates this facet is only slightly bent on itself.

The surface contours of the sacral auricular facet were studied in detail by Weisel using cartographic data, and he has shown (Fig. 16) that it is usually longer and narrower than its iliac counterpart. The sacral facet regularly exhibits the following features:
- a central depression at the junction of its two segments (shown as −)
- two elevations near the extremities of both segments (shown as +).

The iliac auricular facet is reciprocally shortened but without complete symmetry. At the junction of its two segments there is an elevation known as Bonnaire's tubercle. Weisel has also developed a personal theory regarding the arrangement of the sacroiliac ligaments in terms of the forces applied to them. He divides those ligaments into **two groups** (Fig. 17):
- a **cranial group** (arrow Cr), running laterally and posteriorly and counteracting the component F1 of the body weight (P) applied to the superior aspect of S1 (these ligaments are thrown into action by *forward displacement of the sacral promontory*, which is part of the movement of nutation*; see page 63)
- a **caudal group** (arrow Ca) running craniad and opposing the component F2 acting perpendicularly to the superior surface of S1.

* Nutation (Lat: *nutare* = to nod) describes a complex movement of the sacrum analogous to nodding of the head.

Fig. 15

Fig. 16

Fig. 17

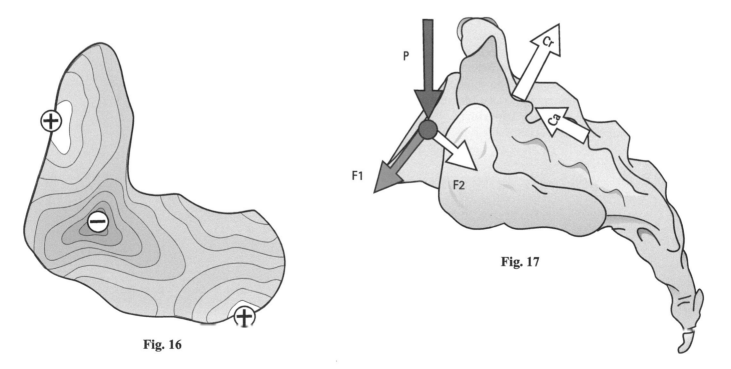

The sacroiliac ligaments

A **posterior view of the pelvis** (Fig. 18) shows the two bundles of the iliolumbar ligament:
- **the superior bundle** (1)
- **the inferior bundle** (2).

On the *right side of the figure* can be seen the intermediate plane of sacroiliac ligaments, which are as follows craniocaudally:
- the **ligament running from the iliac crest to the transverse tubercle of S1** (3)
- the **posterior sacroiliac ligaments** (4) running from the posterior extremity of the iliac crest to the sacral transverse tubercles as follows, according to Farabeuf:
  - the *first* runs from the posterior aspect of the iliac tuberosity to the first sacral tubercle
  - the *second* (also called the ligament of **Zaglas**) is attached to the second tubercle
  - the *third and fourth* run from the posterior superior iliac spine to the third and fourth tubercles.

On the left side of the picture is the **anterior plane of the sacroiliac ligaments** (5), which consists of a fan-shaped fibrous sheet running from the posterior border of the iliac bone to the posteromedial sacral tubercles.

Between the lower part of the external border of the sacrum and the greater sciatic notch there are two *important ligaments:*
- the *sacrospinous ligament* (6), which runs obliquely superiorly, medially and posteriorly from the ischial spine to the lateral border of the sacrum and the coccyx
- the *sacrotuberous ligament* (7), which crosses obliquely the posterior surface of the former. Superiorly it is attached along a line stretching down from the posterior border of the iliac bone to the first two coccygeal vertebrae. Its oblique fibres run a twisting course inferiorly, anteriorly and laterally to be inserted into the ischial tuberosity and the medial lip of the ascending ramus of the ischium. The sciatic notch is thus divided by these two ligaments into **two foramina:**
  - the **greater sciatic foramen superiorly**, which allows the *piriformis muscle* to leave the pelvis

- the **lesser sciatic foramen inferiorly**, through which exits the *obturator internus.*
- an **anterior view** of the pelvis (Fig. 19) shows again the **iliolumbar** (1 and 2), the **sacrospinous** (6) and the **sacrotuberous** (7) ligaments, as well as the **anterior sacroiliac ligament**, consisting of two bundles (also known as the **superior and inferior brakes of nutation):**
  - the **anteroposterior** bundle (8)
  - the **anteroinferior** bundle (9).

Figure 20 shows the **right sacroiliac joint**, opened by rotation of its constituent bones around a vertical axis, and its ligaments. The medial surface of the iliac bone (A) and the lateral surface of the sacrum (B) are exposed, making it easy to understand the following:
- **how the ligaments are wrapped around the joint** and how they become lax or taut during nutation and counternutation
- **why the fibres of the anterior sacroiliac ligament** (8 and 9) **run obliquely inferiorly, anteriorly and medially** from the iliac bone and superiorly, anteriorly and laterally from the sacrum (B).

Also visible in the figure are the following:
- the **posterior sacroiliac ligaments** (5)
- the sacrospinous (6) and the sacrotuberous (7) ligaments
- the **interosseous sacroiliac ligament** (shown as white patches on the two halves of the figure in the concavities of the articular surfaces), which forms the deep layer of the sacroiliac ligaments and is attached laterally to the iliac tuberosity and medially to the anterior foramina of S1 and S2. It is also known as the **axial** or **vague ligament** and is classically considered to represent the axis of movement of the sacrum; hence the term 'axial'.

Fig. 18

Fig. 19

Fig. 20

The legends are the same for all figures.

Nutation and counternutation

Before studying the movements at the sacroiliac joint, it is wise to recall that their range is small and varies according to circumstances and the subject. This explains the contradictions among various authors regarding the function of this joint and the relevance of its movements during labour. These movements were first described by Zaglas in 1851 and by Duncan in 1854.

The classic theory of nutation and counternutation

During the movement of nutation (Fig. 22) the sacrum (red arrow) rotates around an axis (black cross) formed by the **interosseous ligament**, so that its promontory moves **inferiorly and anteriorly** (S2), while its apex and the tip of the coccyx move **posteriorly** (d2).

During this **tilting** motion, which could be compared to the anteroposterior diameter of the pelvic inlet (PI) is reduced by a distance of S2, and the anteroposterior diameter of the pelvic outlet (PO) is increased by a distance d2. At the same time (Fig. 21) the wings of the iliac bones move closer together, while the ischial tuberosities move apart. This movement of nutation is limited (see Fig. 20, p. 59) by the tension developed in the *sacrotuberous* (6) and *sacrospinous* (7) *ligaments* and in the *nutation brakes*, i.e. *the anteroposterior* (8) *and the anteroinferior* (9) *bundles of the anterior sacroiliac ligament.*

A **coronal section of the pelvis** (Fig. 23) shows **the widening of the pelvic inlet** (PI) **and of the pelvic outlet** (PO) during nutation along with the approximation of the iliac crests at the level of the anterior superior iliac spines (asis).

Counternutation (Fig. 25) involves movements in the opposite direction. The sacrum pivots around the interosseous ligament (black cross) and rights itself so that its promontory moves **superiorly and posteriorly** (S1) and its apex and the tip of the coccyx move inferiorly and anteriorly (d1).

As the **sacrum rights itself into counternutation**, the anteroposterior diameter of the pelvic inlet (PI) is increased by a distance of S1 and the anteroposterior diameter of the pelvic outlet (PO) is reduced by a distance of d1. At the same time (Fig. 24) *the wings of the iliac bones move apart and the ischial tuberosities are drawn closer together.*

The movement of counternutation is limited (see Fig. 20, p. 59) by the tension of the anterior (5) and the deep (4) sacroiliac ligaments. As a guideline, the change in the anteroposterior diameter of the pelvic outlet can amount to 3 mm according to Bonnaire, Pinard and Pinzani and to 8-13 mm according to Walcher. The range of the changes in the anteroposterior diameter of the pelvic outlet can amount to 15 mm according to Borcel and Fernstrôm and to 17.5 mm according to Thoms. Weisel has recently confirmed the transverse displacement of the wings of the iliac bones and of the ischial tuberosities.

Fig. 21

Fig. 22

Fig. 23

Fig. 24

Fig. 25

The various theories of nutation

According to **the classic theory of Farabeuf** (Fig. 26), which we have just described, the tilting of the sacrum **R** occurs about an axis formed by the interosseous ligament, its displacement is angular and its promontory moves inferiorly and anteriorly along an arc of a circle with centre (+) located behind the auricular surface.

According to Bonnaire's theory (Fig. 27), the sacrum is tilted about an axis (+) that passes through Bonnaire's tubercle, located at the junction of the two segments of its auricular surface. Thus the centre of this angular movement (R) is intra-articular.

The studies of **Weisel** allow two other possible theories:

- The **theory of pure translation** (Fig. 28, T) states that the sacrum slides along the axis of the caudal segment of the auricular facet. This would mean a linear displacement resulting in a corresponding displacement of the sacral promontory and of the sacral apex.
- The other theory is based on **rotational movement** (Fig. 29, R) around a perpendicular axis lying inferior and anterior to the sacrum. The location of this centre of rotation would vary from person to person, and with the type of movement involved.

The variety of theories available suggests **how difficult it is to analyse** movements of small range and raises the possibility that different types of movement may occur in different individuals. These ideas have more than abstract significance, since **these movements participate in the physiology of labour and thus are important in practice.**

Fig. 26

Fig. 27

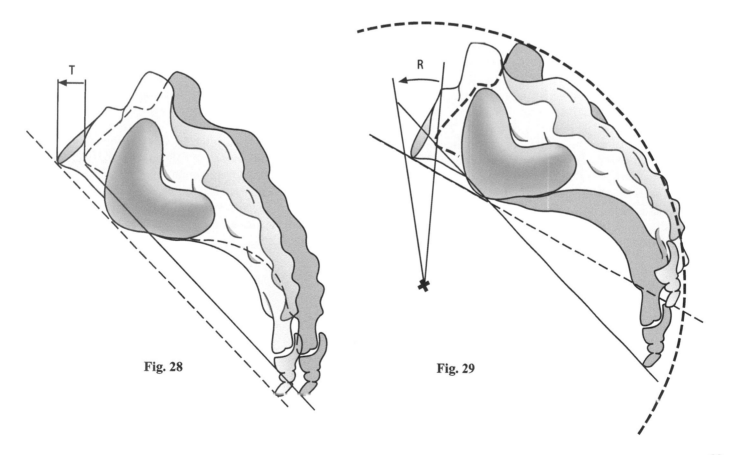

Fig. 28

Fig. 29

The pubic symphysis and the sacrococcygeal joint

The pubic symphysis is an **amphiarthrosis**, i.e. a secondary cartilaginous joint of minimal, if any, mobility. Nonetheless at the end of pregnancy and during labour *water imbibition* by its soft tissues allows the two pubic bones to *slide on each other and move apart.* In rodents these movements have a sizable range. **A horizontal section** (Fig. 30) shows the two medial ends of the pubic bones lined axially by cartilage (10) and united by **the interosseous ligament** (11), a fibrocartilaginous disc with a thin median cleft (12). On the *anterior surface* of the symphysis there is a thic k and predominantly fibrous ligament (7-8-9), whose structure will be presented later. On its *posterior surface* lies the **posterior pubic ligament** (5).

On **a medial view of** the opened joint (Fig. 31, right side) the articular surface of the pubic bone appears oval, with its oblique long axis running superiorly and anteriorly, and is topped by the tendon of origin of the **rectus abdominis** (1). The joint is locked anteriorly by the very thick **anterior pubic ligament** (3), made up of transverse and oblique fibres, as clearly seen in the anterior view (Fig. 34). These fibres consist of the following:

- the aponeurotic insertions of the **external oblique** (8)
- the tendinous origins of the **rectus abdominis** (7) and of the **pyramidalis** (2)
- the tendons of origin of the **gracilis** and of the **adductor longus** (9).

All these fibres crisscross anterior to the symphysis and form a dense fibrous feltwork, the **prepubic ligament.**

The **posterior aspect of the joint** (Fig. 33) bears the **posterior pubic ligament** (5), which is a fibrous membrane continuous with the periosteum. Also visible is a triangular aponeurotic band, whose base rests on the superior borders of the symphysis and of the pubic bones deep to the rectus, and whose oblique fibres are inserted at various levels into the midline of the linea alba. It is known as the **admuniculum lineae albae** (6), i.e. the reinforcement of the linea alba.

A vertical section taken in a coronal plane (Fig. 32) shows the components of the articular surfaces:

- the **hyaline cartilage** lining the pubic bones (10)
- the **fibrocartilaginous disc** (11)
- the **thin cleft** (12) in the fibrocartilaginous disc.

The superior border of the symphysis is strengthened by the **superior pubic ligament** (13), which is a thick and dense fibrous band. The inferior border is strengthened by the **inferior or arcuate** pubic ligament, which is continuous with the interosseous ligament and forms a sharp-edged arch rounding off the apex of the pubic arch. The thickness and strength of the **rib vault of the pubic arch** (4) are clearly seen in the sagittal section (Fig. 31). These powerful periarticular ligaments make the symphysis a *very strong joint that is difficult to dislocate.* In clinical practice traumatic dislocation rarely occurs and is generally difficult to treat when it does occur; this is surprising for a joint that is apparently fixed under normal circumstances.

The **sacrococcygeal joint**, connecting the sacrum and the coccyx, is an **amphiarthrosis.** Its articular surfaces are elliptical, with their long axes running transversely. A **lateral view** (Fig. 37) shows the convex sacral surface and the concave coccygeal surface. The joint is united by an **interosseous ligament** similar to an intervertebral disc and by **periarticular ligaments**, which fall into three groups: anterior, posterior and lateral. The **anterior view** (Fig. 35) shows the **coccyx** (1), which is a *vestigial tail* and is made up of *four fused bony vertebrae*, the **sacrum** (2) and the **anterior ligament**, and on the anterior surface of the sacrum, the vestigial **anterior longitudinal vertebral ligament** (3), which becomes continuous with the **anterior sacrococcygeal ligament** (16). Three **lateral sacrococcygeal ligaments** (5, 6 and 15) can also be seen. The **posterior view** (Fig. 36) shows vestigial ligaments on the **median crest of the sacrum** (13), which are continuous with the **posterior sacrococcygeal ligaments** (14).

At the sacrococcygeal joint the only movements are those of **flexion-extension**, which are only **passive** and occur during *defecation* and *labour.* During nutation of the sacrum the posterior tilting of the sacral apex can be *amplified and extended by extension of the coccyx* inferiorly and posteriorly. This **increases the anteroposterior diameter of the pelvic outlet** during delivery of the fetal head.

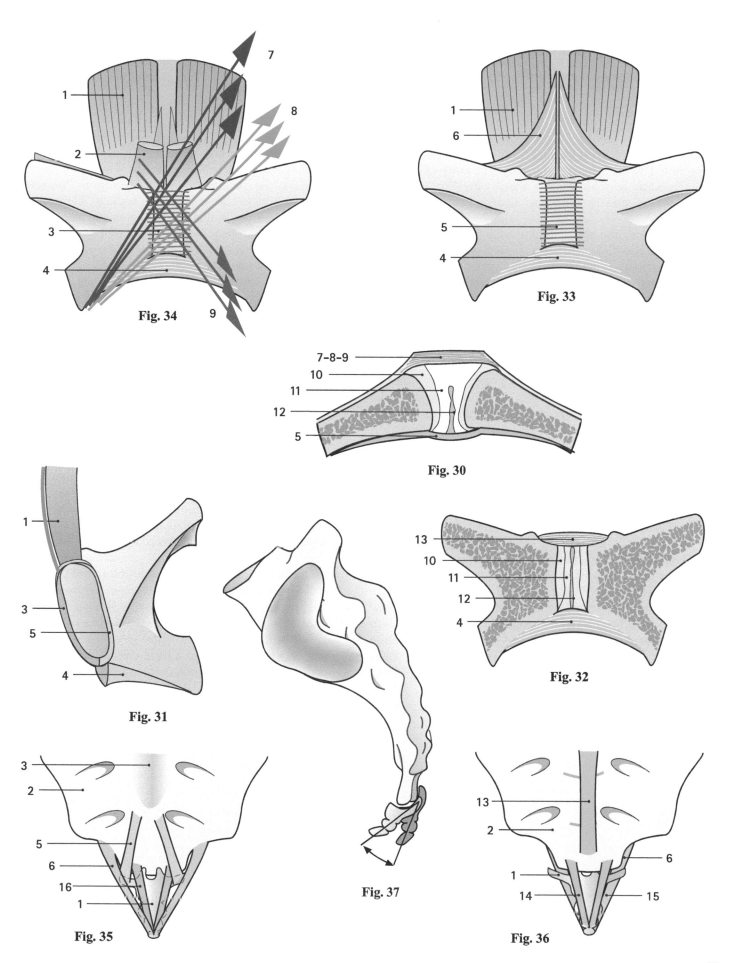

Fig. 34

Fig. 33

Fig. 30

Fig. 31

Fig. 32

Fig. 35

Fig. 37

Fig. 36

65

The legends are the same for all figures.

The influence of position on the joints of the pelvic girdle

In the symmetrical erect posture the joints of the pelvic girdle are recruited by the weight of the body. The mode of action of these forces can be analysed on a lateral view (Fig. 38), where the iliopsoas is considered transparent and allows the femur to be seen.

The vertebral column, the sacrum, the hip bones and the lower limbs form a coordinated articular system with two joints: the hip joint and the sacroiliac joint. The weight of the trunk (P) acts on the sacrum and tends to lower its promontory. The sacrum then undergoes a **movement of nutation** (N2), which is rapidly limited by the anterior sacroiliac ligaments (the **brakes of nutation**), and above all by the **sacrospinous** and the **sacrotuberous ligaments**, thus preventing the sacral apex from moving away from the ischial tuberosity.

At the same time, the **reaction of the ground** (R), transmitted by the femora at the hip joints, forms (with the weight of the body acting on the sacrum) a rotatory couple that causes the hip bone to tilt posteriorly (N1). This retroversion of the pelvis *increases the movement of nutation at the sacroiliac joints*. This analysis deals with movements, but it should rather deal with forces, **because the ligaments are extremely powerful** and stop all movement immediately.

Figure 40 shows that, in the symmetrical erect posture, the **centre of gravity of the body** (G) lies midway on a line joining S3 to the pubis (P) nearly at the **level of the hip joints**, where the pelvis settles into the position of equilibrium.

In the one-legged position (Fig. 39) *at every step taken* the reaction of the ground (R) is transmitted by the supporting limb and elevates the corresponding hip while the other hip is pulled down by the weight of the freely hanging limb (D). This leads to a **shearing force in the pubic symphysis**, which tends to raise the pubic bone on the supporting side (A) and lower the opposite pubic bone (B). Normally the robustness of the symphysis precludes any movement, but, when it is dislocated, the upper borders of the pubic bones become misaligned **m** during walking. In the same way one can imagine **the recruitment of the sacroiliac joints** in the *opposite direction* during walking. Their resistance to movement resides in their *strong ligaments* but, after dislocation of one of the sacroiliac joints, painful movements occur at every step. *Therefore both standing and walking depend on the mechanical robustness of the pelvic girdle.*

In the supine position the sacroiliac joints are recruited differently, depending on whether the hip is flexed or extended.

- **When the hips are extended** (Fig. 41) the pull of the **flexor muscles** (e.g. the psoas visible in the figure) tilts the pelvis anteriorly, while the sacral apex is pushed anteriorly. This shortens the distance between the sacral apex and the ischial tuberosity and rotates the sacroiliac joint into counternutation. This position corresponds to the early stage of labour, and the counternutation, which enlarges the pelvic inlet, favours the descent of the fetal head into the true pelvis.

- **When the hips are flexed** (Fig. 42) the pull on the **hamstrings** (shown in the diagram) tends to tilt the pelvis posteriorly relative to the sacrum, i.e. **a movement of nutation**, which decreases the diameter of the pelvic inlet and increases both diameters of the pelvic outlet. This position, taken during the **expulsive phase of labour**, thus favours the **delivery of the fetal head** through the pelvic outlet.

- During a change of position from hip extension to hip flexion, the mean range of **displacement of the sacral promontory is 5.6 mm.** Therefore these changes in the position of the thighs markedly alter the dimensions of the pelvic cavity in order to facilitate the passage of the fetal head during labour. When the thighs are flexed on the pelvis the lumbar lordosis (Fig. 41) is flattened and a hand can no longer be slipped under the small of the back (green arrow).

Fig. 38

Fig. 39

Fig. 40

Fig. 41

Fig. 42

The pelvic wall

A **medial view of the right hemipelvis** (Fig. 43, after removal of the left hip bone) shows only the right hip bone and the sacrum with two ligaments:
- the sacrospinous ligament (1), which runs from the lateral border of the sacrum to the ischial spine
- the sacrotuberous ligament (2), which runs from the inferior part of the lateral border of the sacrum and of the coccyx to the ischial tuberosity and sends a falciform expansion (3) on to the ischiopubic ramus.

These two ligaments join the hip bone and the sacrum to form the two foramina (i.e. the greater sciatic notch superiorly [s] and the lesser sciatic notch inferiorly [i]). These foramina connect the pelvic cavity to the lower limb.

A **similar medial view of the right hemipelvis** (Fig. 44) also contains two external rotator muscles of the lower limb (see Volume 2) after leaving the pelvis via these two foramina:
- the **piriformis** (4), which arises from the pelvic surface of the sacrum on both sides of the second and third sacral foramina and is inserted into the greater trochanter after passing through the greater sciatic foramen with the gluteal artery above (red arrow) and the sciatic nerve below (yellow arrow)
- the **obturator internus** (5) which arises from the border of the **obturator foramen** (this old name, inherited from the classical authors is an oxymoron, since a hole cannot be closed) and the quadrilateral surface (q)* and bends acutely at the posterior border of the lesser sciatic notch, runs anteriorly and laterally with the gemellus muscles (not seen in the diagram) to be inserted into the greater trochanter. The sciatic artery (red arrow) also exits via the lesser sciatic foramen.

These two muscles are also lateral rotators of the lower limb (see Volume 2).

Another medial view of the right hemipelvis (Fig. 45) now also contains two flexor muscles of the lower limb as they leave the pelvis under the inguinal ligament (il) on top of the horizontal pubic ramus. They are as follows:
- the **iliacus** (6), which has a wide fleshy origin from the entire pelvic surface of the iliac bone
- the **psoas major** (7), which arises from the transverse processes of the lumbar vertebrae.

These two muscles join to form the **iliopsoas** before being inserted by a common tendon into the lesser trochanter.

The osteomuscular pelvic wall (Fig. 46, **medial view**) gives attachment to a very large muscle, the **levator ani** (8), which lies symmetrically on either side of the midline of the **pelvic diaphragm** and arises along a line that borders the pelvic wall, i.e. from the following structures arranged anteroposteriorly:
- the pelvic surface of the pubis (not shown)
- the obturator fascia arching over the obturator foramen
- the tendinous arch of levator ani connecting the external border of the sacrum to the ischial spine
- the pelvic surface of the sacrotuberous ligament
- the lower part of the lateral border of the sacrum and the external border of the coccyx
- the anococcygeal ligament running from the tip of the coccyx to the anus (a).

This wide muscular sheet consists of many bundles well described by anatomists and forms the **pelvic diaphragm, which holds in place and supports all the abdominal and pelvic viscera.** This partition is interrupted of necessity along the midline by **important tubular structures:** two in men (the **anus** and the **urethra**) and yet a third in women (the **vagina**). Here lies the problem of the perineum!

---

* The quadrilateral surface (q) is the pelvic surface counterpart of the iliac bone contribution to the articular and non-articular surface of the acetabulum.

Fig. 43

Fig. 44

Fig. 45

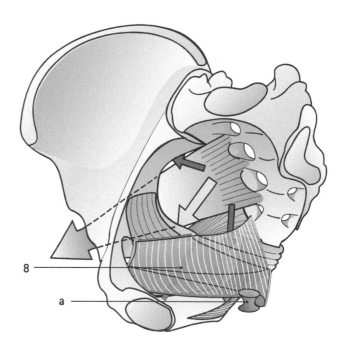

Fig. 46

The pelvic diaphragm

A view of the pelvis taken from behind, below and outside (Fig. 47) clearly shows the wide muscular sheet formed by the various components of the levator ani around the anus **a.**

This muscular diaphragm (Fig. 48) is a perfect *counterpart to the thoracic diaphragm.* It has similar functions (i.e. **separating and retaining the viscera**) and also contains openings for the **passage of important organs.**

Thus in women it contains a large cleft, the **urogenital cleft** (Fig. 49,c). In both sexes, however, the anus, located in its posterior part, is surrounded by a special sling, i.e. the **levator ani** (8), whose fibres blend more or less with those of the anal sphincter and play an important role in the mechanism of *anal continence and defecation.*

A **coronal section** (Fig. 50) shows that this partition is not horizontal but is **oblique** and **funnel-shaped** and open below at the urogenital cleft **c.** Moreover, it is lined by a lower and more superficial **second diaphragm**, i.e. the **perineum** (P), which is horizontal and varies in structure with the sexes.

A **posterior view** (Fig. 51) shows these two planes very well:
- the deep plane: the levator ani with its posterior (8) and anterior (8′) bundles
- the superficial plane: the perineum (P), which is attached laterally to the ischiopubic rami and converges centrally on the anal sphincter (as) and anococcygeal ligament (ac).

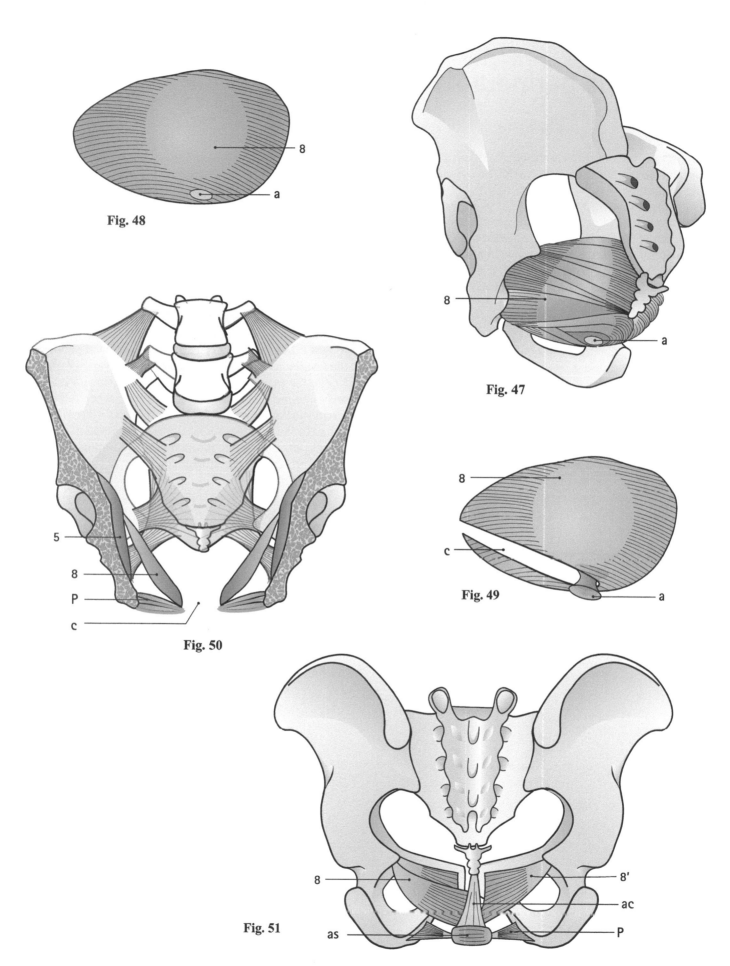

Fig. 48

Fig. 47

Fig. 49

Fig. 50

Fig. 51

71

The female perineum

A left view of the female pelvis (Fig. 52) **taken from behind, below and outside** brings out clearly the *two planes* of the female perineum.

- The **superficial plane** consists of the **superficial transversus perinei** (1) running transversely between the two ischiopubic rami and of two sphincteric muscles, which are circular and can thus control the calibre of an anatomical orifice ; hydraulically it is equivalent to a tap or a sluice. For comparison, the face has a similar muscle, i.e., the orbicularis oris:
  - anteriorly the **sphincter urethrovaginalis** (4) surrounding the vaginal orifice (v)
  - posteriorly the **anal sphincter** (5), which forms a muscular ring around the anus (a).
- The **deep plane** is made up of the following:
  - the **deep transversus perinei** (2), which has the same attachments and course as the anal sphincter
  - the **ischiocavernosus** (seen as transparent, 7) surrounds the corpus cavernosum; it arises from the ischiopubic ramus and meets its counterpart to surround the *clitoris* under the pubic symphysis. Its function is to compress the corpus cavernosum and therefore it lies parallel to it.

- These two planes are separated by the superior and inferior fascial layers of the urogenital diaphragm (3), which extend posteriorly (3′) just beyond the transversus muscles.
- In the centre of this structure all the muscle fibres and their aponeuroses become tightly interwoven to form the perineal body (6), which is a vital element in the robustness of the female perineum. It is prolonged posteriorly by the anococcygeal ligament (8), which connects the tip of the coccyx to the anal sphincter.

All these structures are visible in the **position adopted during a gynaecological examination** (Fig. 53) and can also be seen individually in the diagram drawn in perspective (Fig. 54).

A view taken in perspective of the superficial perineum and the levator ani (Fig. 55) brings out their relationships.

Unlike the male perineum, the female perineum is subject to severe traumas, especially during labour, when the fetus must forcibly make its way through the urogenital cleft, which is supported by the anterior medial fibres of the levator ani (L). These traumas can destabilize the static equilibrium of the pelvis and lead to prolapse of the urogenital organs.

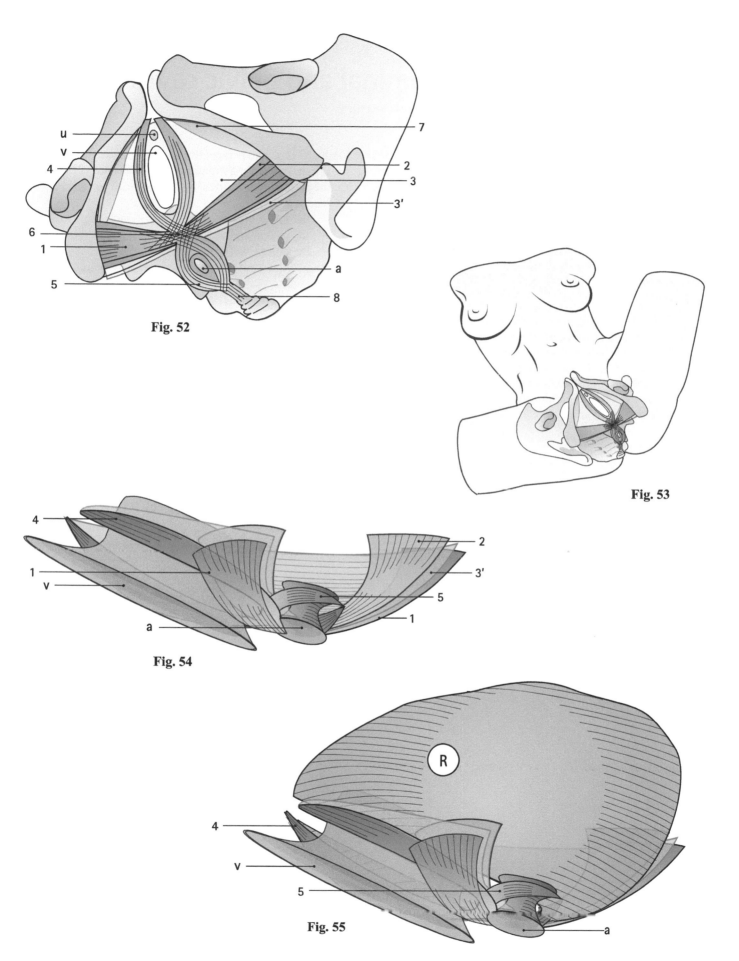

Fig. 52

Fig. 53

Fig. 54

Fig. 55

The volumes of the abdominal and pelvic cavities

An anteroposterior view taken in perspective (Fig. 56) brings out the virtual volume of the combined abdominopelvic cavity. This global volume is divided into two by the pelvic inlet (red), as seen in **a view of these three openings taken in perspective** (Fig. 57).

The pelvic inlet coincides with the pelvic ring. **It is a continuous circular line running from the sacral promontory** (i.e. the projecting anterior border of the upper surface of S1) **to the upper border of the pubic symphysis.** On both sides it crosses the **arcuate line** of the ilium.

The dimensions of these openings are well known and of considerable importance during pregnancy. They can be measured radiographically with relative ease.

Another look at Figure 56 shows that the **volume of the abdomen** (clear and transparent), strictly speaking lying above the pelvic inlet, is clearly greater than that of the **true pelvis,** which lies below (in blue).

Figure 57 (taken in perspective) brings out two other openings of great importance for the passage of the fetal head during labour:
- the **intermediate opening** (green line) demarcated by four landmarks:
  - the lower border of the pubic symphysis
  - the ischial spines
  - the pelvic surface of the sacrum
- the **pelvic outlet** (dotted blue line), also demarcated by four landmarks:
  - the lower border of the pubic symphysis
  - the tip of the coccyx
  - the pelvic surfaces of the ischial tuberosities.

As the term fetus shifts from its abdominal to its pelvic location, on its way out, it enters the so-called **birth canal** (Fig. 58), which can be conceptualized by an anteriorly concave large tube passing through all three straits.

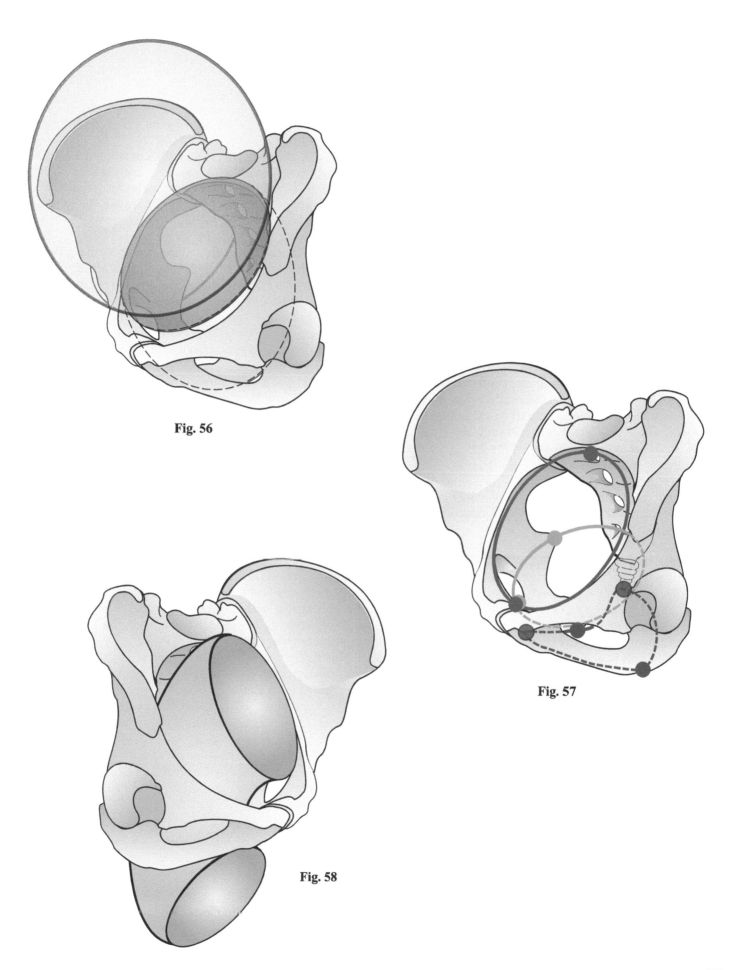

Fig. 56

Fig. 57

Fig. 58

Labour

This is not an obstetrics textbook and there is no intention of describing in detail the mechanisms of normal labour, and even less of abnormal labour.

This physiological process, however, is of interest here insofar as it depends on the **locomotor apparatus in its broad sense**, i.e. the skeleton, the joints and muscles of the abdomen and pelvis.

At term, pregnancy is followed by **labour**, i.e. the expulsion of the fetus **per vias naturales.** It must be stressed that the delivery of the fetus is **a natural physiological process**, which has occurred over the aeons to ensure the survival of the human race. Thus obstetrics is the science of the mechanisms of normal and abnormal labour, culminating in what is called a 'happy event'.

At the start of labour the entire body of the mother is called to '**action stations**', and the passage of the fetus through the birth canal is the result of a well-coordinated succession of processes. First (Fig. 59) the abdominal muscles **contract to push** the *fetal head through the pelvic inlet*, so that it becomes **engaged** in the true pelvis. The supine position with lower limbs lying flat (see Fig. 41, p. 67) favours the opening of the pelvic outlet via the mechanism of **counternutation.**

The powerful uterine muscle (Fig. 60), made up of *circular, oblique and longitudinal fibres*, starts to contract **rhythmically** and the cervical os begins to dilate. The contractions signal the onset of **labour.**

The increase in the pelvic diameters is facilitated by the widening of the pubic symphysis (Fig. 62).

The hormonal status at the end of pregnancy leads to softening of the pubic symphysis and allows the pubic bones to move apart by 1 cm, thus increasing pelvic diameters, starting with that of the pelvic inlet. When the cervical os is fully dilated, expulsion begins, and there is a need to increase further the diameter of the pelvic outlet. This is achieved by the mechanism of **nutation**, which, as we have already seen, is enhanced by flexion of the thighs on the pelvis (see Fig. 42, p. 67).

The ancestral position for labour, still used by a large portion of humanity, is that of **hanging by the arms** (Fig. 63): hip flexion **promotes nutation** and thus opening of the pelvic outlet; the vertical position enhances the **abdominal thrust**, which results from the weight of the viscera, **the downward displacement of the diaphragm and contraction of the abdominal muscles** (Fig. 61). The most effective muscles in this process are not the straight muscles but rather the large flat muscles, such as the external and internal oblique muscles and especially the **transversus abdominis**, which bring back towards the spine and the **axis of the birth canal** the now grossly enlarged uterus as it tilts forwards over the pubic symphysis.

Recent publications by the well-known obstetrician Bernadette de Gasquet have shown the important role of certain positions of the hips and especially of the femurs in making delivery easier. She has shown that medial or lateral rotation of the femurs has a profound effect on the geometry of the bony pelvis and so on the dimensions of the pelvic inlet and of the pelvic outlet, which need to be crossed successively during delivery.

During the first phase ('labour period'), lateral rotation of the femurs (Fig. 62bis, red arrows around the femurs) produces counternutation that, by modifying the tension in some muscles and ligaments, tends to cause the iliac bone to tilt laterally (upper blue arrows), widening the pelvic inlet through the backward displacement of the sacral promontory (upper central blue arrow) and favouring the passage of the infant's head into the lesser pelvis.

In contrast, during the second phase ('delivery period'), medial rotation of the femurs (Fig. 63bis, red arrows around the femurs) produces nutation through the opposite effect on the muscles and ligaments: the iliac wings are drawn closer together (upper green arrows), most notably the ischial tuberosities move apart (lower little green arrows) and the iliac bone moves backwards, thereby widening the pelvic outlet and favouring expulsion of the foetus. Medial rotation of the femurs is easy to achieve by moving the legs outwards with respect to the knees, which are taken to be fixed; likewise, moving the legs towards the midline produces lateral rotation of the femurs.

This method is used more and more, and by shortening the time of delivery reduces the degree of foetal distress and the pain of expelling the foetus.

The anatomical and functional characteristics of the female perineum set the stage for functional disorders caused by *ageing* and by *multiple pregnancies* in some women. The urogenital cleft then provides a possible path for the descent of the pelvic viscera, e.g. the bladder, the urethra and the uterus, resulting in **urogenital prolapse.**

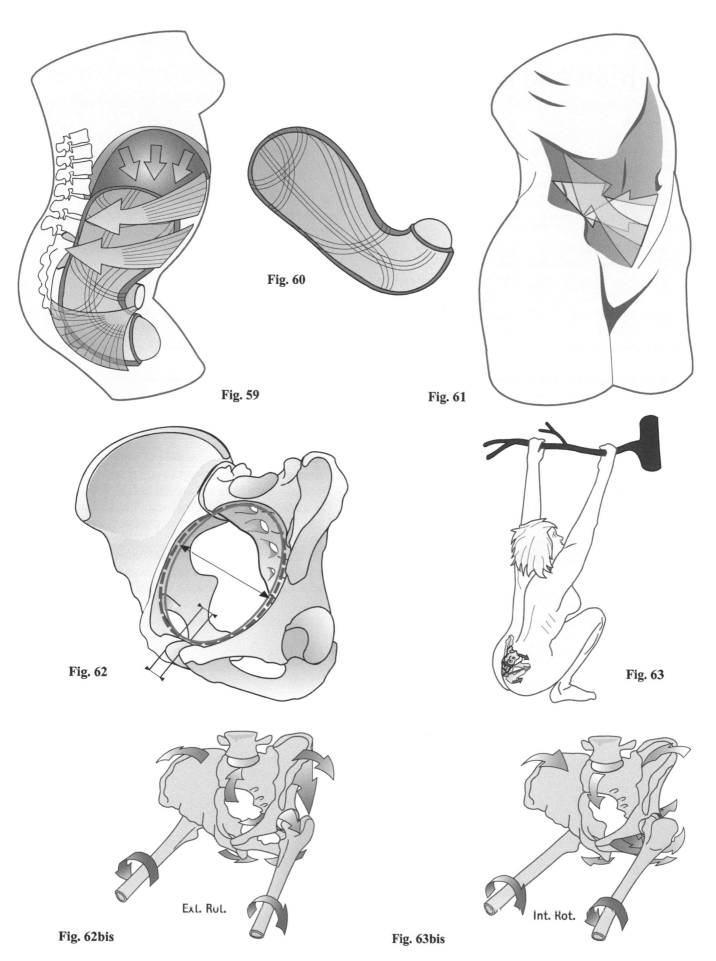

Fig. 60

Fig. 59

Fig. 61

Fig. 62

Fig. 63

Ext. Rot.

Fig. 62bis

Int. Rot.

Fig. 63bis

Micturition and defecation in the female

The perineal muscles control essential processes like **micturition, defecation** and **erection.**

Let us look at the role of the female perineum in micturition and defecation, which occur in both sexes. First we shall consider the mechanisms of urinary continence and micturition.

The control of urination

The bladder is a **reservoir** that accommodates the *continuous formation of urine by the kidneys* and allows the sporadic passage of urine at will. Bladder filling triggers the desire to void. **Urinary continence** and **voluntary control of urination** are vital for the autonomy of the individual.

Urinary continence in women (Fig. 64) allows the progressive filling of the bladder (b), which is the most anterior organ in the pelvis. As long as the **internal urethral sphincter** (1), which consists of smooth muscle, remains contracted, there is no leakage of urine. The **external urethral sphincter** (2), which consists of voluntary striated muscle, lies in the superficial plane of the perineum downstream from the internal sphincter. It is the voluntary contraction of the external sphincter that *prevents micturition* in the presence of a very strong urge to urinate at an ill-timed moment.

Micturition (Fig. 65) (i.e. urination or satisfying the need to urinate) depends on four mechanisms:

- the relaxation of the **involuntary** internal urethral sphincter
- contraction of the **detrusor**, a smooth muscle in the bladder wall
- relaxation of the external urethral sphincter
- contraction of the muscles underlying the **abdominal effort** during micturition, i.e. the diaphragm (d) and the broad abdominal muscles, especially the internal oblique (5) and the transversus (6).

The control of defecation

Faeces accumulate in the rectum, which is the large-calibre terminal portion of the sigmoid colon. When the rectum (r) is filled, the desire to defecate is felt.

Faecal continence (Fig. 66) is controlled by the action of two muscles:

- the **levator ani** (3), whose deepest fibres crisscross the anal canal posteriorly and contract to bend the anal canal at an acute angle by pulling it forwards
- the **external anal sphincter** (4), which consists of voluntary striated muscle and lies in the superficial plane of the perineum downstream from the internal anal sphincter; its contraction controls faecal retention and its relaxation controls defecation.

Defecation (Fig. 67) or the release of faecal material depends on four mechanisms:

- relaxation of the levator ani (3), which allows the canal to become once more straight and vertical
- contraction of the smooth muscles of the rectal wall (r), especially the longitudinal and circular bundles, in a peristaltic fashion, i.e. waves of repeated contractions moving downstream
- relaxation of the external anal sphincter (4)
- contraction of the abdominal muscles, contributing to the abdominal effort during defecation, i.e. the diaphragm (d) and the broad muscles of the abdomen, especially the external oblique (5) and above all the transversus (6).

Fig. 64

Fig. 65

Fig. 66

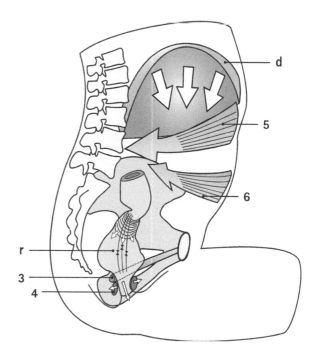

Fig. 67

The legends are the same for all figures.

The male perineum

Unlike the female perineum the male perineum is straightforward, i.e. no delivery, no prolapse and no urinary incontinence, except postoperatively. On the other hand, men are prone to urinary retention because of *prostatic disease*.

Anatomically the **male perineum** (Fig. 68) has the *same structural components* as the female perineum, but there is a crucial difference, i.e. there is *no urogenital cleft*.

The male perineum consists of two planes:
- the deep **transversus perinei** (1)
- the superficial **transversus perinei** (2).

These planes are separated by the following:
- the **intermediate perineal ligament** (3), which fills the entire anterior triangle of the perineum
- the **anal sphincter** (4) attached to the coccyx by the **anococcygeal ligament** (5)
- the **external urethral sphincter** (6).

All these structures meet in the midline in **the perineal body** (7). The urogenital cleft is replaced by the erector apparatus made up of **three erectile bodies**, which act as sponges and can swell with blood supplied by the **pudendal arteries.** Along the ischiopubic rami are also found the two **corpora cavernosa** (8), which are surrounded by the **ischiocavernous muscles** (9) and meet in the midline below the pubic symphysis to form the *dorsal part of the penis.*

As the **urethra** (u) traverses the perineum it is embedded in the **corpus spongiosum** (10), which is surrounded by the **bulbospongiosus** (11) and is slung by the perineal ligament as it courses along the midline towards the confluence of the cavernosa to contribute to the formation of the **penis** (p). These three erectile bodies are surrounded by the **inextensible deep fascia of the penis**, which acts as a sheath contributing to the erection of the penis. The male urethra ends at the external urinary meatus at the tip of the glans.

Urinary control (Fig. 69) depends on the same structures as in women, but with an additional structure, the prostate (P). This gland lies at the base of the bladder and surrounds the urethra; its function is to secrete seminal fluid, which keeps the spermatozoa in suspension.

Normally when the **bladder** fills up two sphincters ensure continence:
- the **involuntary internal urethral sphincter** (2), which surrounds the first part of the prostatic urethra
- the **voluntary external urethral sphincter** (3), which lies at the prostatic apex and ensures *voluntary urinary control.*

When there is *nodular prostatic hyperplasia* the enlarged prostate projects into the first part of the prostatic urethra and hinders the emptying of the bladder, which then dilates from urinary retention and extends as a dome (d, dotted line) above the pubis. **Micturition** (Fig. 70) results from contraction of the **detrusor**, while the **internal** (2) **and the external** (3) **urethral sphincters** relax. No abdominal effort is usually necessary except when there is urinary retention.

Erection, *which renders the penis rigid*, is easy to understand with the use of a novelty party hooter. This is a tubular paper ribbon, closed at one end and fitted with a spring that allows it to roll up on itself (Fig. 71). When one blows into it (Fig. 72) through its open end it swells up, gets longer and becomes rigid. During erection the corpora cavernosa and corpus spongiosum swell up like the ribbon and become rigid because of the inflow of blood from the pudendal arteries while the venous outflow is obstructed.

An **experimental demonstration** of this process can be carried out with a rubber fingerstall (or a condom) attached to a base with an inflow tap and an outflow tap (Fig. 73). When the inflow tap is closed, corresponding to the closure of the pudendal veins, blowing into the inflow tap causes the fingerstall to swell. If, in addition, the fingerstall is tightened at its base (Fig. 75), simulating the contraction of the ischiocavernosus and of the bulbospongiosus, its volume and rigidity are increased. It is the spasm of the ischiocavernosus and bulbospongiosus that sets the time of **ejaculation** by vigorously ejecting the spermatozoa lying in the urethra and leads to **orgasm.** The pleasure of orgasm is the 'reward' to the individual for performing the basic act that will ensure his continuation via the act of procreation. Continued involuntary penile erection is **priapism**, which is a very painful condition.

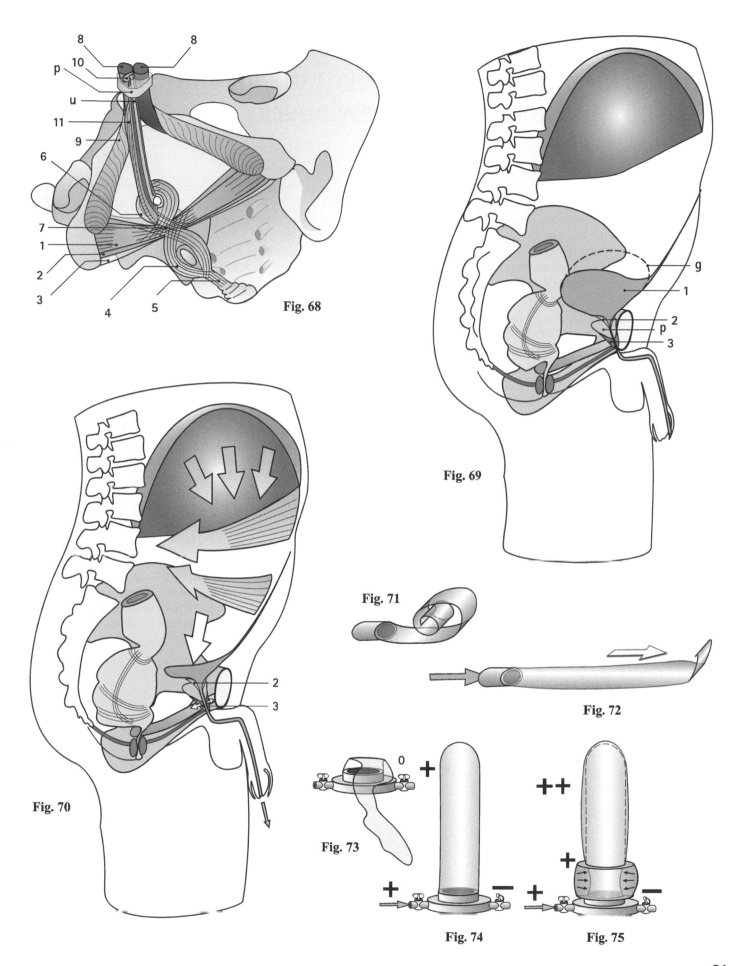

Fig. 68

Fig. 69

Fig. 70

Fig. 71

Fig. 72

Fig. 73

Fig. 74

Fig. 75

External landmarks of the pelvis: the lozenge of Michaelis and the plane of Lewinneck

Besides more or less sophisticated radiological examinations, a simple clinical examination using posterior and anterior landmarks can help understand the structure of the pelvis.

The human back (Fig. 76) **has the easily detected midline spinal furrow**, which lies between the paravertebral muscles and corresponds to the interspinous line. It stops at the bottom at the level of the sacrum, where the **lozenge of Michaelis** stands out with its four apices:

- on either side of the midline, the **two sacral fossae**
- above, the **lower extremity of the spinal furrow**
- below, the **summit of the natal cleft.**

Thus the lozenge has a **vertical long axis** in the midline continuous with the spinal groove and a **short transverse axis**, perpendicular to the former and running between the sacral fossae. The *length of the short axis* is constant, whereas *that of the long axis* varies so that the lozenge appears more or less flattened depending on the individual.

Since the classical period of Greek history, *sculptors and painters* have always included this lozenge in their works, as can be observed on all their *paintings and sculptures*. Some modern artists know the name, but among doctors only obstetricians are familiar with this name. This is not by chance, since **Gustav Adolph Michaelis** (1798-1848) was a German gynaecologist who lived in Kiehl *before radiography was available*. He discovered the lozenge as a means of recognizing *possible pelvic deformities that could lead to dystocia*. **Radiography** has made it possible to know what structures correspond to the lozenge.

Anterior views (Fig. 77), using lead markers (small white circles) to identify the four apices, show the following correlations:

- the apices corresponding to the two **sacral fossae** that contain the lateral lead markers always overlie the **upper part of the sacroiliac joints**

- the position of the superior apex varies between **L4** and **L4–L5**
- the inferior apex can also oscillate slightly about its projection on **S3**.

This lozenge lies in a region of great aesthetic value, hence its name of '*divine lozenge*'. It corresponds to the sacrum and to the lumbosacral junction and is of considerable interest to surgeons and rheumatologists.

In fact, three landmarks help to demarcate this **lumbosacral region** (Fig. 78):

- **the space between the spines of L4 and L5,** where the intercristal line (between the iliac bones) crosses the midline
- the **two sacral fossae**, where injections can be made into the sacroiliac joints
- the **first superior posterior sacral foramen**, through which it is easy to administer **low peridural injections**, e.g. into the sciatic nerves. It lies (dark blue) *two finger breadths below L4-L5* and *two finger breadths away from the midline*. Once the *superficial tissues have been patiently anaesthetized* it becomes easy to look for this sacral foramen with a fairly long needle, and it is reached when the needle has lost contact with the sacral bone and one gets the impression of no resistance. The needle is then pushed carefully in for 1 cm and the injection can begin.

On the anterior surface of the pelvis (Fig. 79) the two anterior superior iliac spines and the pubic crest demarcate the **triangle of Lewinneck**, which supports the pelvis in the **prone position** (Fig. 80). This triangle is a stereotactic landmark for computer-guided operations on the pelvis.

Fig. 76

Fig. 77

Fig. 78

Fig. 79

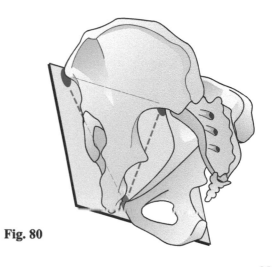

Fig. 80

Chapter 3

THE LUMBAR SPINE

The lumbar spine rests on the pelvis and articulates with the sacrum. In turn it supports the thoracic spine, which is linked to the thorax and the scapular girdle.

Next to the cervical spine the lumbar spine is the **most mobile segment** and also **bears the brunt of the weight** of the trunk.

As a result, it is the main seat of disease, including the most common of all skeletal disorders, **lumbago**, secondary to **herniation of the intervertebral disc.**

Global view of the lumbar spine

An **anteroposterior** radiograph (Fig. 1) shows that the lumbar spine is **straight and symmetrical** relative **to the interspinous line** (m). The width of the vertebral bodies and that of their transverse processes *decreases regularly* craniad. The **horizontal line** (h), passing through the highest points of the two iliac crests, runs between L4 and L5. The vertical lines (a and a′), drawn along the lateral borders of the sacral alae, run roughly through the **floor of each acetabulum.**

An **oblique view** (Fig. 2) illustrates the components of the **lumbar lordosis** and the static features of the lumbar spine, as worked out by de Sèze:

- the **sacral angle** (a), formed between the horizontal and the line passing through the upper border of S1, averages 30°
- the **lumbosacral angle** (b), formed between the axis of L5 and the sacral axis, averages 140°
- the **angle of inclination of the pelvis** (i), formed between the horizontal and the line joining the sacral promontory to the superior border of the pubic symphysis, averages 60°

- the **arc of the lumbar lordosis** can be completed by a line joining the posterosuperior border of L1 to the posteroinferior border of L5, and corresponding (p) to the chord of the arc (c, orange-dashed line). The perpendicular (p) to the chord is usually longest at the level of L3. It increases as the lordosis is more marked and almost disappears when the lumbar spine is straight. It can rarely become inverted
- the **posterior bend** (indicated by arrow pb) represents the distance between the posteroinferior border of L5 and the vertical line passing through the posterosuperior border of L1, and can be:
  - **zero** if the vertical line coincides with the chord of the lumbar lordosis
  - **positive** if the lumbar spine is bent backward
  - **negative** if the lumbar spine is bent forward.

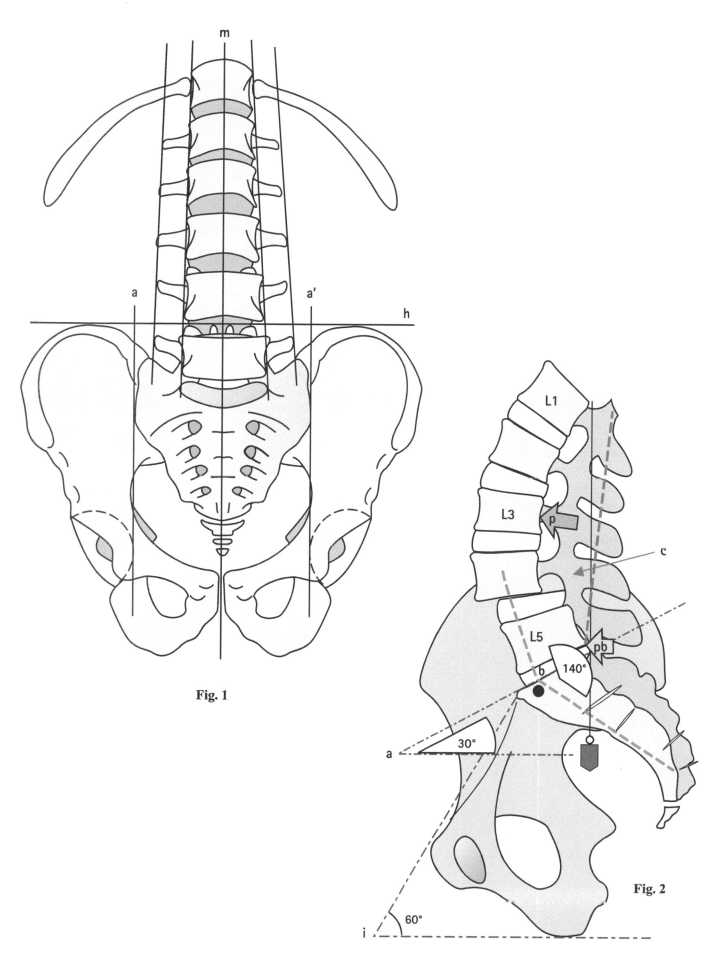

Fig. 1

Fig. 2

Structure of the lumbar vertebrae

A '**disassembled**' **view** (Fig. 3) brings out the components of the lumbar vertebra:

- **The kidney-shaped vertebral body** (1) is wider laterally than it is deep anteroposteriorly, and is broader than it is high. Its periphery is deeply hollowed out in the shape of a *diabolo*, except posteriorly, where it is nearly flat.
- **The two laminae** (2) are quite tall and run posteriorly and medially, and they lie in a plane that is oblique inferiorly and superiorly.
- The bulky and rectangular **spinous process** (3), formed in the midline by fusion of the two laminae, runs backwards into a bulbous tip.
- The **transverse processes** (4), better called the *costoid processes*, are in fact vestigial ribs attached at the level of the articular processes and running an oblique course posteriorly and laterally. On the posterior aspect of their site of attachment lies the *accessory process* (not shown), which, according to some authors, is the homologue of the transverse process of a thoracic vertebra.
- The **pedicle** (5) is a short bony segment joining the vertebral arch to the vertebral body and is attached to the former at its superolateral angle. It defines the superior and inferior limits of the adjacent intervertebral foramen and posteriorly provides attachment for the **articular processes.**
- The **superior articular process** (6) lies on the upper border of the lamina as it joins the pedicle. It lies in a plane running obliquely, posteriorly and laterally, and its cartilage-coated **articular surface** faces posteriorly and medially.
- The **inferior articular process** (7) arises from the inferior border of the vertebral arch near the junction of the lamina with the spinous process. It faces inferiorly and medially, and its cartilage-coated **articular surface** faces *laterally and anteriorly.*
- The **vertebral foramen** lies between the posterior surface of the vertebra and the vertebral arch in the shape of an *almost equilateral triangle.*

The **typical lumbar vertebra** is 'reassembled' in Figure 4.

Some lumbar vertebrae have certain specific features. The transverse process of L1 is *less well developed* than those of the other lumbar vertebrae. The vertebral body of L5 is *higher anteriorly than posteriorly*, so that its profile is **wedge-shaped** or even trapezoidal, with its longer side lying anteriorly. Its inferior articular surfaces are more widely separated from each other than those of the other lumbar vertebrae.

When *two lumbar vertebrae are separated vertically* (Fig. 5) it becomes obvious how the inferior articular processes of the upper vertebra **fit snugly,** medially and posteriorly into the superior articular process of the lower vertebra (Fig. 6). Thus each lumbar vertebra *stabilizes* the overlying vertebra *laterally* **as a result of the lateral buttress-like structure of the articular processes.**

Fig. 3

Fig. 4

Fig. 5

Fig. 6

The ligamentous complex of the lumbar spine

This ligamentous complex can be studied, on the one hand, on a **sagittal section** (Fig. 7, after removal of the laminae on the left) and, on the other, on a **coronal section** (Fig. 8, passing through the pedicles and containing the vertebral bodies seen from the back). The **posterior half of the section** (Fig. 9), after a rotation of 180°, contains the vertebral arches seen from the front and a detached vertebra lying on top. Note that in Figures 8 and 9 the corresponding stumps of the pedicles are seen on both sides.

The sagittal section (Fig. 7) reveals very clearly two sets of ligaments:

- the **anterior** (1) **and posterior** (5) **longitudinal ligaments** running along the entire spine
- the **segmental ligaments running between the vertebral arches.**

The **anterior longitudinal ligament** (1) stretches as a long, thick, pearly band from the basilar process of the occipital bone to the sacrum on the anterior surfaces of the vertebrae. It consists of long fibres running from one end of the ligament to the other and short arcuate fibres bridging the individual vertebrae. It is inserted into the **anterior aspect of the intervertebral disc** (3) and into the **anterior surface of the vertebral body** (2). Thus, at the anterosuperior and anteroinferior angles of each vertebra there are **two potential spaces** (4), where **osteophytes** (bony outgrowths) are formed in vertebral osteoarthritis.

The **posterior longitudinal ligament** (5) extends from the basilar process of the occipital bone to the sacral canal. Its two edges are *festooned* because its **arcuate fibres** (6) are inserted a long way laterally into each intervertebral disc. On the other hand, the ligament is *not attached to the posterior surface of the vertebra*, leaving a space (7) traversed by *paravertebral venous plexuses*. The concavity of each festoon corresponds *to a pedicle* (10).

The sagittal section (Fig. 7) shows the intervertebral disc with its **annulus fibrosus** (8) and its **nucleus pulposus** (9).

Segmental ligaments bind the **vertebral arches**. Each lamina is joined to the next by a thick powerful yellow ligament, the **ligamentum flavum** (11), seen transected in Figure 7. It is inserted inferiorly into the superior border of the underlying lamina and superiorly into the medial aspect of the overlying lamina. Its medial edge fuses with that of the contralateral ligament in the midline (Fig. 9) and completely closes the **vertebral canal posteriorly** (13). Anteriorly and laterally it overlies the capsular and **anteromedial ligaments** (14) of the facet joints. Thus its anteromedial border is flush with the *posterior margin of the intervertebral foramen*.

The spinous processes (12) are linked by the powerful **interspinous ligaments** (15), continuous posteriorly with the **supraspinous ligaments** (16), which are attached to the *tips of the spinous processes*. In the lumbar region the ligaments are indistinct as they merge with the crisscrossing fibrous attachments of the lumbodorsal muscles.

The **intertransverse ligaments** (17), well developed in the lumbar region, run on both sides between the accessory processes of the adjacent transverse processes.

On an **anterior view of the vertebral arch** (Fig. 9), cutting through the *ligamentum flavum* (13) has allowed the upper vertebra to be detached; between C2 and C3 the ligament has been completely resected to reveal the capsule, the **anteromedial ligament of the facet joint** (14) and the spinous process between the two vertebral arches.

Taken together, these two sets of ligaments form an **extremely strong link** between the two vertebral bodies and also for the spine as a whole. Only a *severe trauma* can break this link.

Fig. 7

Fig.8

Fig. 9

The legends are the same for all figures.

Flexion-extension and lateral flexion of the lumbar spine

During flexion (Fig. 10) the body of the upper vertebra tilts and glides slightly forward in the direction of the arrow F, reducing the thickness of the intervertebral disc anteriorly and increasing it posteriorly. Thus the disc becomes wedge-shaped, with its base facing posteriorly, and the nucleus pulposus is driven posteriorly, stretching the posterior fibres of the annulus fibrosus.

At the same time the inferior articular processes of the upper vertebra glide upwards and tend to free themselves from the superior articular processes of the lower vertebra (black arrow). As a result the capsule and the ligaments of this facet joint are maximally stretched along with the other ligaments of the vertebral arch – the ligamentum flavum, the interspinous ligament (2), the supraspinous ligament and the posterior longitudinal ligament. The tension of these ligaments finally limits extension.

During extension (Fig. 11) the body of the upper vertebra tilts and moves posteriorly in the direction of the arrow E. Meanwhile, the disc becomes flatter posteriorly and thicker anteriorly and is transformed into a wedge with its base lying anteriorly. The nucleus is pushed anteriorly, stretching the anterior fibres of the annulus and the anterior longitudinal ligament (4). On the other hand, the posterior longitudinal ligament is relaxed, the articular processes of the upper and lower vertebrae become more tightly interlocked (3) and the spinous processes touch each other. Hence extension is limited by the impact of the bony structures of the arch and by the stretching of the anterior longitudinal ligament.

During lateral flexion (Fig. 12) the body of the upper vertebra tilts on the side of flexion (arrow 1), while the disc becomes wedge-shaped and thicker on the other side, with displacement of the nucleus. The contralateral intertransverse ligament (6) is stretched, while the ipsilateral ligament (7) slackens (see Fig. 13).

A posterior view (Fig. 13) shows how the articular processes glide relative to each other: the articular process of the upper vertebra is raised on the convex side (8), while it is lowered on the concave side (9). This leads at the same time to relaxation of the ipsilateral ligamenta flava and of the capsular ligament of the facet joint and to the stretching of the same structures contralaterally.

Fig. 10

Fig. 11

Fig. 12

Fig. 13

Rotation in the lumbar spine

A superior view (Figs 14 and 15) shows the *superior articular facets* of the lumbar vertebrae facing **posteriorly and medially**. They are not flat but *concave transversely and straight vertically*. Geometrically speaking, they correspond to segments of a cylinder with centre O located posteriorly **near the base of the spinous process** (Fig. 16).

In the case of the **upper lumbar vertebrae** (Fig. 14) the centre O of this cylinder lies just behind the line joining the posterior borders of the articular processes, whereas for the **lower lumbar vertebrae** (Fig. 15) the diameter of this cylinder is much greater, so that its centre O lies far more posteriorly.

It must be stressed that *the centre of this cylinder does not coincide with the centres of the vertebral discal surfaces*, so that, when the upper vertebra rotates on the lower vertebra (Figs 18 and 19), the rotational movement occurring around this latter centre has to be associated **with a gliding movement of the upper vertebra** relative to the lower vertebra (Fig. 16). Thus the disc D is not only rotated axially (Fig. 17) – which would allow a relatively much greater range of movement – but is also subject to gliding and shearing movements (Fig. 16). As a result, axial rotation of the lumbar spine is quite limited both segmentally and globally. According to Gregersen and Lucas, axial rotation of the lumbar spine between L1 and S1 would have a total range bilaterally of 10° and so a segmental range of 2° (assuming equal segmental distribution) and a segmental range of 1° for unilateral rotation. It becomes obvious that the lumbar spine is **not at all designed for axial rotation**, which is sharply limited by the orientation of the vertebral articular facets.

Fig. 14

Fig. 15

Fig. 16

Fig. 17

Fig. 18

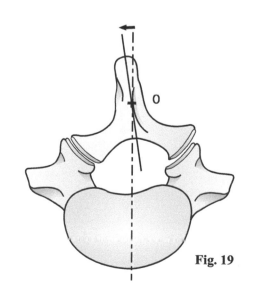

Fig. 19

The lumbosacral hinge and spondylolisthesis

The lumbosacral hinge is **a weak point in the spine**.

A **lateral view** (Fig. 20) shows that, as a result of the inclination of the upper surface of S1, the body of L5 tends to glide inferiorly and anteriorly. The weight (P) can be resolved into two elementary forces:

- a force (N) acting perpendicular to the upper surface of S1
- a force (G) acting parallel to the upper surface of S1 and pulling L5 anteriorly.

This gliding movement is prevented by the powerful anchoring of the vertebral arch of L5.

A **superior view** (Fig. 22) shows the inferior articular processes of L5 fitting tightly into the superior articular processes of S1. The gliding force (G′) presses the articular processes of L5 hard against the superior articular processes of the sacrum, which react with a force R on both sides.

These forces are **by necessity transmitted through a single point in the vertebral isthmus** or pars interarticularis (Fig. 21), which is the part of the vertebral arch lying between the superior and inferior articular processes. When this isthmus is fractured or destroyed, as shown here, the condition is known as **spondylolysis.** As the arch is no longer retained posteriorly on the superior articular processes of the sacrum, *the body of L5 glides inferiorly and anteriorly* giving rise to **spondylolisthesis.** The

only structures that still retain L5 on the sacrum and prevent further slippage are:

- the **lumbosacral intervertebral disc**, whose oblique fibres are stretched
- the **paravertebral muscles**, which go into permanent spasm and cause the pain associated with spondylolisthesis.

The degree of slippage can be measured anteriorly by the degree of overhanging of L5 relative to the anterior border of the upper surface of S1.

Radiographs taken from an oblique view (Fig. 23) reveal the classic picture of the 'Scottie dog':

- its muzzle corresponds to the transverse process
- its eye to the pedicle seen head-on
- its ear to the superior articular process
- its front paw to the inferior articular process
- its tail to the lamina and the contralateral superior articular process
- its hind paw to the contralateral inferior articular process
- its body to the lamina on the same side as the picture is taken.

The important point is that *the neck corresponds exactly to the vertebral isthmus*. When **the isthmus is broken, the neck of the dog is transected,** clinching the **diagnosis of spondylolisthesis.** Anterior slippage of L5 must then be looked for in oblique views.

Fig. 20

Fig. 21

Fig. 22

Fig. 23

The iliolumbar ligaments and movements at the lumbosacral hinge

An anterior view of the lumbosacral hinge (Fig. 24) shows the last two lumbar vertebrae united directly to the hip bones by the **iliolumbar ligaments**, made up of the following:

- **the superior band** (1), attached to the tip of the transverse process of L4 and running inferiorly, laterally and posteriorly to be inserted into the iliac crest
- **the inferior band** (2), attached to the tip and lower border of the transverse process of L5 and running inferiorly and laterally to be inserted into the iliac crest *anteromedially to the superior band.*

Sometimes two more or less distinct bands can be made out:

- a strictly **iliac** band (2)
- a **sacral** band (3), which runs more *vertically* and slightly anteriorly and is inserted distally into the anterior surface of the sacroiliac joint and into the most lateral part of the sacral ala.
- These two iliolumbar ligaments are tightened or slackened depending on the movements at the lumbosacral hinge and thus help limit these movements as follows:
- **During lateral flexion** (Fig 25) the iliolumbar ligaments become taut contralaterally and allow only an 8° movement

of L4 relative to the sacrum. The ipsilateral ligaments are slackened.

- **During flexion-extension** (Fig. 26, lateral view with the iliac bone transparent) starting from the neutral position **N**:
  - the direction of the ligaments is responsible **during flexion** (F) for the selective *tightening of the superior band of the iliolumbar ligament* (red), which runs an oblique course inferiorly, laterally and posteriorly. Conversely, this band is relaxed **during extension** (E)
  - on the other hand, *the inferior band of the iliolumbar ligament* (blue) is slackened **during flexion** (F) as it runs slightly anteriorly and is stretched **during extension** (E).

On the whole, mobility at the lumbosacral joint is sharply limited *by the strength of the iliolumbar ligaments.* All things considered, **they limit lateral flexion much more than flexion-extension.**

1

2

3

Fig. 24

8°

Fig. 25

F N E

Fig. 26

The trunk muscles seen in horizontal section

Figure 27 shows the inferior aspect of a horizontal cross-section passing through L3. **Three muscle groups** can be identified. **The posterior paravertebral muscles can be subdivided into three planes.**

1. The **deep plane**, comprises the following:
- the **transversospinalis** (1), which fills up the solid angle between the sagittal plane of the spinous processes and the coronal plane of the transverse processes and is closely moulded onto the vertebral laminae
- the **longissimus** (2), which overlies the former and over-extends it laterally
- the **erector spinae** (3), a bulky fleshy muscle lying lateral to the former
- finally the **interspinalis** (4) attached to the spinous processes and lying posterior to the transversospinalis and the longissimus.

These muscles form a large fleshy mass that lies on both sides of the spinous processes in the paravertebral gutters; hence their name of paravertebral muscles. They are separated externally by the **lumbar furrow**, which corresponds to the **interspinous line**.

2. The **intermediate plane**, consisting of the **serratus posterior superior and serratus posterior inferior** (5).

3. The **superficial plane**, consisting in the lumbar region of only one muscle, the **latissimus dorsi** (6), which arises from the very thick lumbar fascia (7) partly attached to the interspinous line. The **body of the muscle** (6) forms a thick fleshy carpet over the *whole of the posterolateral wall of the lumbar region*.

The deep lateral paravertebral muscles are two in number:
- the **quadratus lumborum** (8), which is a muscular sheet attached to the last rib, the transverse processes of the lumbar vertebrae and the iliac crest
- the **psoas** major (9), which is a very long muscle, lying within the solid angle formed by the lateral borders of the vertebral bodies and the transverse processes.

The muscles of the abdominal wall fall into two groups:
- the **rectus abdominis muscles** (13) lying on both sides of the midline
- the **large abdominal muscles**, which form the *anterolateral wall of the abdomen* and are, from deep to superficial, the **transversus abdominis** (10), the **internal oblique** (11) and the **external oblique** (12).

Anteriorly these muscles form aponeurotic insertions that give rise to the **rectus sheath** and the **linea alba** as follows.
- The aponeurosis of the internal oblique *splits at the lateral border of the rectus* to form two fascial sheets, one **deep** (14) and the other **superficial** (15), which enclose the rectus. The sheets *crisscross* in the midline to form a very *solid raphe* – the **linea alba** (16).
- The anterior and posterior sheets of the rectus sheath are reinforced posteriorly by the *aponeurosis of the transversus* and anteriorly by the *aponeurosis of the external oblique*. This only applies to the upper part of the abdomen; we shall see later exactly what happens in the lower part.
- The deep lateral paravertebral muscles and the large abdominal muscles bound the **abdominal cavity**, into which project the **lumbar spine** and the **large paravertebral vessels**, i.e. the aorta and the inferior vena cava (not shown here).
- The **true abdominal cavity** (18) is bounded and lined by the **parietal peritoneum** (21) (red), which also lines the posterior aspect of the rectus muscles, the deep aspects of the large abdominal muscles and the posterior abdominal wall, to which are attached the retroperitoneal organs, e.g. the kidneys, embedded in the **retroperitoneal space** (19), which is made up of loose areolar fat. Between the parietal peritoneum and the abdominal wall lies a thin fibrous layer, i.e. the **fascia transversalis** (17).

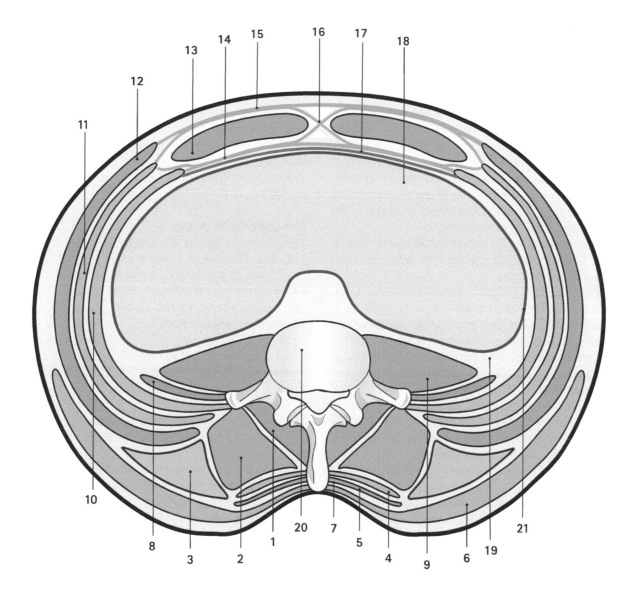

Fig. 27

The posterior muscles of the trunk

These posterior muscles are arranged in three planes from deep to superficial.

The deep plane

The deep plane consists of the spinal muscles directly attached to the vertebrae (Figs 28 and 29); hence their name of **paravertebral muscles.** *The deeper they lie, the shorter the course of their fibres.*

- The **transversospinalis** (1) is made up of lamellae arranged like tiles on a roof. In the diagram (inspired by Trolard), where only one set of lamellae is included, the oblique fibres run inferiorly and laterally from the lamina of one vertebra to the transverse processes of the four underlying vertebrae. According to Winckler, the fibres run from the laminae and the spinous processes of a set of four upper vertebrae to the transverse process of the lower vertebra.
- The **interspinalis muscles** (2) connect the adjoining spinous processes on both sides of the midline. The diagram shows only one set of these muscles.
- The fusiform **spinalis** (3), lies on either side of the interspinalis muscles and posterior to the transversospinalis. It arises inferiorly from the upper two lumbar vertebrae and from the last two thoracic vertebrae and is inserted above into the spinous processes of the first 10 thoracic vertebrae. The deepest fibres run the shortest course.
- The **longissimus thoracis** (5) is a long muscle lying lateral to the spinalis. It runs in the posterior wall of the thorax to be inserted into the lower 10 ribs (its lateral or costal fibres) and into the transverse processes of the lumbar and thoracic vertebrae (its medial or transverse fibres).
- The **thoracic part of the iliocostalis** (6) is a thick muscle mass in the shape of a prism. It lies posterior and lateral to the above-mentioned muscles. It runs in the posterior wall of the thorax, giving off branches to be inserted into the posterior surfaces of the lower 10 ribs near their posterior angles. These fibres are then relayed by the fibres of the longissimus cervicis, which run upwards to the transverse processes of the last five cervical vertebrae (see 11, Fig. 95, p. 259).

In the lower part of the trunk all these muscles intermingle to form **a common body of lumbar muscles** (6), seen on the right of Figure 29. These are inserted into the deep aspect of a thick tendinous sheath, which is continuous superficially with the **aponeurosis of the latissimus dorsi** (7).

The intermediate plane

This plane (Fig. 29) comprises a single muscle, i.e. the **serratus posterior inferior** (4), lying immediately behind the paravertebral muscles and in front of the latissimus dorsi. It arises from the spines of the *first three lumbar and last two thoracic vertebrae* and runs obliquely superiorly and laterally to be inserted into the lower borders and external aspects of the last three or four ribs.

The superficial plane

This plane consists of the **latissimus dorsi** (7) (see Volume 1, p. 73, Fig. 115), which arises from the very thick lumbar aponeurosis. Its oblique tendinous fibres run superiorly and laterally on top of all the paravertebral muscles and give rise to muscular fibres along an oblique line running inferiorly and laterally.

The **lumbar aponeurosis** as a whole forms a *lozenge with a vertically oriented long axis.* The muscle fibres give rise to a broad sheet *covering the posterolateral part of the lower thorax* on their way to their insertion into the humerus.

The action of the posterior muscles is essentially an **extension of the lumbar spine** (Fig. 30). From their sacral anchor they can powerfully pull *backwards* the lumbar and thoracic segments of the spine at the lumbosacral hinge and at the thoracolumbar hinge, respectively.

Furthermore they **accentuate the lumbar lordosis** (Fig. 31), since their chords span the full extent or part of the arc of the lumbar curvature. It is incorrect to say that they straighten the lumbar spine; they only pull it posteriorly by bending it. We shall see later that these muscles play an active role in expiration.

Fig. 28

Fig. 29

Fig. 30

Fig. 31

The role of the third lumbar and twelfth thoracic vertebrae

A. Delmas has brought to light the functional significance of certain vertebrae (Figs 32 and 33) in maintaining the erect position. The wedge shape of L5, which acts as a bridge between the more or less horizontal sacrum and the vertical spine, is well known. Conversely, the role of **L3** is just starting to be appreciated (Fig. 32). This vertebra has a *better developed posterior arch*, since it acts as a relay station between the following muscles:

- on the one hand **the lumbar fibres of the longissimus thoracis** muscles, which run from the hip bone to the transverse processes of L3
- on the other hand **the fibres of the interspinalis thoracis** muscles, which arise further up the thoracic spine and are inserted as low as the spinous process of L3.

Thus (Fig. 33: the spinal column, shown in profile), L3 is *pulled posteriorly by muscles attached to the sacrum and the ilium* to provide a locus for the action of the thoracic muscles. Therefore it plays the essential role of *pivot vertebra* and **relay station** for the spine at rest, the more so as it coincides with the apex of the lumbar curvature and its horizontal superior and inferior surfaces are parallel to each other. It is the first truly mobile lumbar vertebra, since L4 and L5, strongly bound to the ilium and the sacrum as they are, form a bridge more static than dynamic between spine and pelvis.

Conversely, the **twelfth thoracic vertebra** (T12) is *the point of inflexion between the thoracic and lumbar curvatures*. It acts as a **hinge vertebra**: its body is relatively important with respect to its posterior arch, which lies in front of the paravertebral muscles as they course along without inserting. Delmas considers T12 as '*the true swivel of the vertebral axis*'.

Fig. 32

T12

L3

Fig. 33

The lateral muscles of the trunk

They are two in number: the quadratus lumborum and the psoas major.

The quadratus lumborum (Fig. 34, anterior view), as its name implies, forms a *quadrilateral* muscular sheet. It spans the last rib, iliac crest and spine, and has a free lateral border. It is made up of three sets of fibres (right side of figure):

- fibres running *directly* between the last rib and the iliac crest (orange arrows)
- fibres running between the last rib and the transverse processes of the five lumbar vertebrae (red arrows)
- fibres running between the transverse processes of the first four lumbar vertebrae and the iliac crest (green arrows). These fibres are continuous with those of the transversospinalis (violet arrows), which lie in the spaces between the transverse processes.

These three sets of fibres of the quadratus are also arranged in three planes – the posterior plane consisting of the straight iliocostal fibres, the intermediate plane of the iliovertebral fibres and the anterior plane of the **costovertebral fibres** (1). When the quadratus **contracts unilaterally** it bends the trunk on the same side (Fig. 35) with considerable help from the internal and external oblique muscles.

The **psoas major** (Fig. 36, 2) lies anterior to the quadratus, and its fusiform muscle belly originates from two separate muscular sheets:

- a **posterior sheet** (Fig. 34, green arrows) attached to the transverse processes of the lumbar vertebrae
- an **anterior sheet** (Fig. 34, blue arrows) attached to the bodies of T12 and L1-L5.

These latter fibres are attached to the lower and upper borders of two adjacent vertebrae and to the lateral border of the intervertebral disc. Tendinous arches bridge over these muscle attachments. The fusiform body of the muscle, flattened anteroposteriorly, runs an oblique course inferiorly and laterally, follows the edge of the pelvic inlet, is *reflected on the anterior edge of the hip bone* and is inserted *along with the iliacus* into **the tip of the lesser trochanter.**

If its femoral insertion is fixed and the hip is stabilized by contraction of the other periarticular muscles, the psoas **exerts a very powerful action on the lumbar spine** (Fig. 37), leading to *lateral flexion ipsilaterally and rotation contralaterally.* Furthermore (Fig. 38), as it is attached to the summit of the lumbar curvature, it also **flexes the lumbar spine** on the pelvis while **increasing the lumbar curvature**, as is clearly seen in a subject lying supine with the lower limbs resting on the underlying surface (Fig. 41, p. 67).

On the whole, the two lateral muscles cause *lateral flexion of the trunk* on the side of their contraction, but, whereas the quadratus has no effect on the lumbar lordosis, the psoas major on the other hand *increases it while rotating the spine contralaterally.*

Fig. 34

Fig. 36

Fig. 35

Fig. 38

Fig. 37

The muscles of the abdominal wall: the rectus abdominis and transversus abdominis

The rectus abdominis

The two rectus muscles (Fig. 39, anterior view and Fig. 40, side view) form *two muscular straps* in the anterior abdominal wall on either side of the midline.

They are inserted into the *anterior arches and costal cartilage of the fifth, sixth and seventh ribs and into the xiphoid process.* Below its insertion the muscle narrows gradually and is interrupted by *tendinous insertions*: two above the umbilicus, one at the level of the umbilicus and one below the umbilicus. Thus the rectus is *polygastric.* Its infra-umbilical part is clearly narrower as it tapers down into its *strong tendon of origin*, which is attached to the upper border of the pubic bone and to the pubic symphysis, and sends slips to *the contralateral muscle and the thigh adductors* (Fig. 43, p. 69).

The rectus muscles are separated by a wider gap across the midline above than below the umbilicus – the **linea alba.** They lie inside the **rectus sheath**, which is formed by the aponeurotic insertions of the large muscles of the abdominal wall (see p. 100).

The transversus abdominis

The two transverse muscles (Fig. 41, anterior view, with only the left transversus included; Fig. 42, side view) form the *deepest layer* of the large muscles of the abdominal wall. They arise posteriorly from the *tips of the transverse processes of the lumbar vertebrae.*

The *horizontal* fibres run laterally and anteriorly around the abdominal viscera and give rise to aponeurotic fibres along a line parallel to the lateral border of the rectus muscles. This aponeurotic insertion joins the *contralateral aponeurosis on the midline*. It lies mostly deep to the rectus abdominis and contributes to the formation of the posterior layer of the rectus sheath, but *below the umbilicus* it runs superficial to the rectus, which *perforates* it so as to gain access to its deep surface. Below this level, which is indicated on the deep surface of the rectus by the **arcuate line** of the rectus sheath, the aponeurosis now contributes to the anterior layer of the rectus sheath.

In the diagram it is clear that only the middle fibres of the aponeurosis are horizontal; the upper fibres run a slightly oblique course superiorly and medially, while the lower fibres run a slightly oblique course inferiorly and medially. The lowermost fibres terminate on the *superior border of the pubic symphysis and of the pubis* and join *those of the internal oblique* to form the **conjoint tendon.**

Fig. 39

Fig. 40

Fig. 41

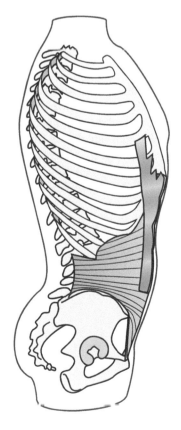

Fig. 42

The muscles of the abdominal wall: the internal and external oblique muscles

The internal oblique muscle of the abdomen

This muscle (Figs 43 and 44) makes up the *intermediate layer* of the abdominal muscles and runs generally speaking an oblique course *superoinferiorly and lateromedially* to the *iliac crest*. Its fleshy fibres provide a muscular sheet on the lateral wall of the abdomen:

- some are inserted directly into the *eleventh and twelfth ribs*
- others indirectly by an aponeurosis into a line that runs first horizontally from the apex of the eleventh rib and then vertically along the lateral edge of the rectus.

These aponeurotic fibres are inserted into the *tenth costal cartilage* and *the xiphoid process*. They contribute to the *anterior layer of the rectus sheath* and, as a result, they blend with similar fibres from the contralateral muscle in the midline to form the *linea alba*.

The lowest fibres of the internal oblique are attached *directly* to the lateral part of the inguinal ligament. They are first horizontal and then oblique inferiorly and medially. They join the transversus abdominis to form the **conjoint tendon** before gaining attachment to the **superior border of the pubic symphysis** and the **pubic crest.** The conjoint tendon thus forms the border of the *deep inguinal ring* along with the medial part of the inguinal ligament.

The external oblique muscle of the abdomen

This muscle (Figs 45 and 46) forms the *superficial layer* of the large muscles of the abdomen and its bunches are visible in well-muscled individuals. Its fibres generally run an oblique course *superoinferiorly and lateromedially*. Its fleshy digitations, arising from *the last seven ribs*, overlap one another inferosuperiorly and *blend with the digitations of the serratus anterior.*

Its muscle bundles form part of the abdominal wall and give rise to an *aponeurosis* along a line of transition, which is at first vertical and parallel to the lateral border of the rectus and then oblique inferiorly and posteriorly. This aponeurosis contributes to the anterior layer of the rectus sheath and blends with its contralateral counterpart along the midline to form the **linea alba.**

The fibres arising from the ninth rib are attached to the *pubic bone* and send *aponeurotic expansions towards the ipsilateral and contralateral adductors of the thigh*. The fibres arising from the tenth rib terminate on the *inguinal ligament*. These two tendinous structures demarcate *the superficial inguinal ring*, which is a triangular opening with its apex facing superolaterally and its inferomedial base constituted by the pubis and the pubic crest, where the **inguinal ligament** is inserted. This account of the abdominal wall muscles forming the anterior group of motor muscles of the spine makes two important points:

- The rectus muscles, lying anteriorly in the abdominal wall, form two muscle bands, which **act at a considerable distance from the spine** between the base of the thorax anteriorly and the pelvic girdle anteriorly. As a result, they are the most efficient flexors of the trunk.
- The large muscles are arranged in three layers with their fibres crisscrossing as in an organized tissue: in the deep layer they run *transversely* as the transversus; in the intermediate layer they are *oblique superiorly and medially* as the internal oblique; and in the superficial layer they are *oblique inferiorly and medially* as the external oblique. In addition to their role in flexion and rotation, they are important in **supporting** the viscera.

Fig. 43

Fig. 44

Fig. 45

Fig. 46

The muscles of the abdominal wall: the curve of the waist

The fibres of the large muscles and their aponeuroses are woven together into **an unbroken girdle around the abdomen** (Fig. 47). In fact the fibres of the external oblique on one side are directly continuous with the fibres of the internal oblique on the other side and vice versa, so much so that, taken globally, the oblique muscles form a weft, which is not rectangular but **diamond-shaped**, i.e. **cut on the bias** in the language of seamstresses. This arrangement allows the weft to adapt to the curve of the waist: one can even say that this **'bias' literally causes the hollow of the waist.** This can easily be demonstrated on a **model:**

- If strings or elastic bands are drawn between two circles (Fig. 48) parallel to the axis uniting the centres of the circles, a *cylindrical surface* is obtained.
- If the upper circle is rotated around the supporting axis that links the centres of the two circles relative to the lower circle (Fig. 49), the strings remain taut but run obliquely so that the envelope of the surface generated is a **solid hyperboloid** bounded on each side by a *hyperbolic curve.*

This mechanism explains readily why the waist is hollow, the more so as the oblique fibres are under stronger tension and the *subcutaneous fat is thinner.* Therefore, the curve of the waist can be restored by **rebuilding the tonus of the oblique abdominal muscles.**

Moreover, the curve of the lower part of the abdomen also depends on the large muscles, which **form a complete abdominal strap** (Fig. 50) or a 'belly band'. The efficiency of this strap depends not so much on the tonus of the rectus muscles as of the *large muscles:*

- the external oblique (transparent green)
- above all the internal oblique (blue)
- even more the lower part of the **transversus** (yellow).

These muscles are very important during the **pushing phase of labour.**

Fig. 47

Fig. 48

Fig. 49

Fig. 50

The muscles of the abdominal wall: rotation of the trunk

Rotation of the spine is produced by the *paravertebral muscles* and the *large muscles of the abdomen.*

The **superior view** of two lumbar vertebrae (Fig. 51) shows that unilateral contraction of the paravertebral muscles produces only a weak rotation, but the deepest muscle layer – the **transverso-spinalis** (TS) – is more effective. With a foothold on the transverse processes of the lower vertebra, it pulls the spinous process of the upper vertebra laterally and produces rotation on the side opposite its contraction around a centre of rotation lying at the base of the spinous process (black cross).

During rotation of the trunk (Fig. 52) the oblique muscles of the abdomen play an essential role. Their mechanical efficiency is enhanced by their spiral *course around the waist* and by *their attachments to the thoracic cage at a distance from the spine,* so that both the lumbar and lower thoracic spines are recruited. To rotate the trunk to the left (Fig. 52) both the *right external oblique* (EO) and *the left internal oblique* (IO) must contract. It is noteworthy that these two muscles are wrapped around the waist in the same direction (Fig. 53) and that their muscular fibres and their aponeuroses are **continuous in the same direction.** They are therefore **synergistic** for this movement of rotation.

Fig. 51

EO

IO

Fig. 52

Fig. 53

The muscles of the abdominal wall: flexion of the trunk

The muscles of the abdominal wall are **powerful flexors of the trunk** (Fig. 54). Lying *anterior to the axis of the spine* they pull the entire spine forward at the *lumbosacral and thoracolumbar hinges*. Their **great strength** relies on the use of the *two long lever arms*:
- the **lower lever arm** corresponds to the distance between the sacral promontory and the pubic symphysis
- the **upper lever arm** corresponds to the distance between the thoracic spine and the xiphoid process. It is represented in the diagram by the triangular bracket, which rests on the thoracic spine and corresponds to the thickness of the lower thorax.

The **rectus abdominis** (RA), which links the xiphoid process directly to the pubic symphysis, is a powerful flexor of the spine and is helped by the internal oblique (IO) and the external oblique (EO), which link the lower border of the thoracic cage to the pelvic girdle. Whereas the rectus acts as a *straight brace, the internal oblique acts as an oblique brace oriented inferiorly and posteriorly, and the external oblique as an oblique brace oriented inferiorly and anteriorly*. These oblique muscles also act as *stays* depending on their degree of obliquity.

These three muscles have a double action:
- on the one hand, they flex the trunk forward (F)
- on the other, they strongly straighten the lumbar lordosis (R).

Fig. 54

The muscles of the abdominal wall: straightening of the lumbar lordosis

The extent of the lumbar lordosis depends not only on the tone of the abdominal and paravertebral muscles but also on *some lower limb muscles* attached to the bony pelvis.

In the **'asthenic'** posture (Fig. 55) the relaxation of the abdominal muscles (blue arrows) *accentuates all three spinal curvatures*:

- the **lumbar lordosis** (L)
- the **thoracic kyphosis** (T)
- the **cervical lordosis** (C).

As a result, the head moves forward (b), the pelvis **tilts anteriorly** (white arrow) and the line joining the anterior superior and the posterior superior iliac spines *becomes oblique inferiorly and anteriorly.*

The **psoas major** (P), which flexes the spine on the pelvis and **accentuates the lumbar lordosis**, becomes hypertonic and aggravates this deformity. This asthenic stance is often seen in people without energy or willpower.

Similar changes in the spine also obtain in women in *late pregnancy,* when the *mechanics of the pelvis and of the spine is considerably disturbed* by the stretching of the abdominal wall muscles and by the forward displacement of the body's centre of gravity by the developing fetus.

Straightening of the spinal curvatures, i.e. corresponding to the **'sthenic'** posture (Fig. 56), starts at the *level of the pelvis.*

The **anterior tilt of the pelvis** is corrected by the **extensor muscles of the hip:**

- As the **hamstrings** (H) and the **gluteus maximus** (G) contract, they tilt the pelvis posteriorly and restore the interspinous line to the horizontal plane. The sacrum also becomes vertical, and this reduces the lumbar curvature.
- The most crucial muscles in reversing the lumbar hyperlordosis are the abdominal muscles, in particular the **rectus muscles** (RA), which act via two long lever arms on the sternum at the level of the xiphoid process and on the pelvis at the level of the pubis.

Therefore the bilateral contraction of the gluteus maximus and of the rectus is needed to **straighten the lumbar curvature.**

From this point onwards the **lumbar paravertebral muscles** (S), as they contract to extend the spine, can pull back the first lumbar vertebra:

- contraction of the dorsal thoracic muscles **flattens the thoracic curvature**
- likewise, the *cervical paravertebral muscles*, as will be discussed later, **flatten the cervical curvature.**

On the whole, the curvatures are flattened and the spine **grows longer** (h) by 1-3 mm (corresponding to a slight increase in the Delmas index).

This is the classic theory, but 'inclinometric' studies (Klausen 1965) indicate that the spine behaves globally like the *shaft of a crane* with a forward cantilever. Simultaneous electromyographic recordings of the posterior trunk muscles and of the abdominal muscles (Asmussen & Klausen 1962) reveal that in 80% of subjects the standing posture, maintained subconsciously by postural reflexes, depends only on the tonic activity of the posterior trunk muscles. When the subject loads the upper part of the spine by placing a weight on the head or carrying weights with hands along the trunk, the cantilever is bent forward slightly, while the lumbar curvature is flattened and the thoracic curvature increases. At the same time the paravertebral muscles increase their tone to counteract the cantilever effect. Therefore the abdominal muscles do not control the subconscious static behaviour of the spine but are recruited when the **lumbar curvature is consciously straightened**, e.g. when standing to attention or cantilevering heavy loads.

Fig. 56

Fig. 55

The trunk as an inflatable structure: the Valsalva manoeuvre

When the trunk is flexed forward (Fig. 57) the stresses on the lumbosacral discs are considerable.

In fact, the weight of the upper trunk and the head acts through the **partial centre of gravity** (P) located just anterior to T12. This weight (P1) is applied at the extremity of the long arm of a lever with its fulcrum at the level of the nucleus pulposus L5-S1. To counterbalance this force, the spinal muscles S1, acting on the short arm of the lever seven to eight times shorter than the long arm, must develop a force of seven to eight times greater than P1. This force acting on the lumbosacral disc is equal to P1 + S1 and increases with *the degree of flexion* or with *the amount of weight carried in the hands.*

To lift a 10-kg weight, with knees flexed and trunk vertical, the force S1 exerted by the spinal muscles is **141 kg.** Lifting the same weight, with extended knees and **trunk bent forward**, requires a force of **256 kg.** If this same weight is carried **with the arms outstretched forward**, the force S1 equals **363 kg.** At this moment the force acting on the nucleus pulposus would be **282-726 kg** and even up to **1200 kg**, this latter value **clearly exceeding the force needed to crush the intervertebral discs**, i.e. *800 kg before age 40 and 450 kg in the aged.*

This *apparent contradiction* can be explained in two ways:

- Firstly, the full impact of the force acting on the disc is *not borne only by the nucleus pulposus*. By measuring intra-nuclear pressures, Nachemson has shown that, when a force is applied to the disc, the *nucleus supports 75% of the load* and the annulus 25%.
- Secondly, the **trunk intervenes globally** (Fig. 58) to relieve the pressure applied to the lumbosacral and lower lumbar intervertebral discs with the help of the **Valsalva manoeuvre**, which consists of **closing the glottis** (G) and **all the abdominal openings** (F) from the anus to the bladder sphincter. This turns the abdominothoracic cavity into a **closed cavity** (A + T), in which the sustained **contraction of the expiratory muscles** and particularly of the **abdominal muscles**, including the rectus abdominis (RA), raises the pressure and transforms it into a **rigid beam** lying *anterior to the spine* and transmitting the forces on to the pelvic girdle and the perineum.

This mechanism, also known as the 'abdominal effort', is used by weightlifters and reduces the pressure on the discs by 50% on the **T12–L1 disc** and **30% on the lumbosacral disc.** For the same reason, the force exerted by the spinal muscles S2 is reduced by 55%.

Although very useful to relieve the pressures applied to the spine, it can only be used for a short time because it requires **complete apnoea**, which leads to significant circulatory disturbances:

- **cerebral venous hypertension**
- **decrease in cardiac venous return**
- **decreased alveolar capillary blood flow**
- **increased pulmonary vascular resistance.**

It also presupposes that the muscles of the abdominal girdle are intact and that the glottis and the abdominal openings can be closed.

Venous return to the heart is shunted into the **vertebral venous plexuses**, thereby increasing the pressure in the cerebrospinal fluid. Therefore, the lifting of heavy loads can only be **short and intense.**

To reduce the pressure on the intervertebral discs it is preferable to **lift weights with the trunk vertical** rather than flexed forward with a large cantilever effect. **This is the advice that must be given to people at risk for disc prolapse.**

A variant of the Valsalva manoeuvre (Fig. 59), used by divers to balance the pressure on either side of the tympanic membrane, consists of **closing the mouth and nostrils** (N) by pinching them and not closing the glottis, which would increase the intracavitary pressure. Swallowing at the same time opens the Eustachian tube (E), increasing the pressure in **the middle ear to balance the external pressure exerted on the eardrum.**

Fig. 57

Fig. 58

Fig 59

The statics of the lumbar spine in the standing position

When the body is **symmetrically** supported on both lower limbs the **side view of the lumbar spine** (Fig. 60) shows a curvature with posterior concavity, called the **lumbar lordosis** (L). In this position the lumbar spine is straight as seen from the back (Fig. 61), but **in one-legged standing** with asymmetrical support (Fig. 62) the spine becomes *concave on the side of the supporting limb* because the pelvis (P) is tilted so that the supporting hip is higher than the resting hip.

To offset this lateral flexion of the lumbar spine, the *thoracic spine is flexed in the opposite direction*, i.e. towards the resting limb and the line passing through the shoulders (Sh) slopes towards the side of support.

Finally, the **cervical spine** shows a curvature concave on the side of support, i.e. similar to that of the lumbar curvature.

In the symmetrical standing position (Fig. 61) the intershoulder line (Sh) is horizontal and parallel to the pelvic line (P) passing through the always clearly visible sacral fossae.

Brügger's electromyographic studies have revealed that during **flexion** of the trunk (Fig. 63), the **thoracic** (Th) **spinal muscles** are the first to contract strongly, followed by the **glutei** (G) and finally the **hamstrings** (H) and the **triceps surae** (T, not shown). At the end of flexion the spine is passively stabilized only by the **vertebral ligaments** (L), fixed as they are to the pelvis, whose anterior tilting is checked by the **hamstrings** (H).

During straightening of the trunk (Fig. 64) the muscles are recruited in inverse order, i.e. first the **hamstrings** (H), then the **glutei** (G) and finally the **lumbar** (L) and **thoracic** (Th) **spinal muscles.**

In the erect position (Fig. 60) the slight tendency to sway forward is offset by the tonic contraction of the posterior muscles of the body, i.e. the **triceps surae** (T), the **hamstrings** (H), the **glutei** (G), the **thoracic** (Th) and the **cervical** (C) **spinal muscles.** Conversely, the abdominal muscles relax (Asmussen). Occasionally one can see on beaches young girls in the **asthenic stance** (Fig. 65) similar to that previously described in men (see Fig. 55, p. 119). The relaxed abdominal muscles allow the belly to protrude (1), the chest is flattened (2) and the head is bent forward (3). All the spinal curvatures are exaggerated: the small of the back is hollow because there is lumbar hyperlordosis (4), the back is humped because the thoracic kyphosis (5) is accentuated and the nape of the neck (6) is hollow because of cervical hyperlordosis. Here again there is a simple remedy: increase muscle tone! Contract the hamstrings, tighten the buttocks, retract the shoulders by pulling on the back muscles and look straight at the horizon… No flaccidity!

Fig. 60

Fig. 61

Fig. 62

Fig. 63

Fig. 64

Fig. 65

The sitting and asymmetrical standing positions: the musician's spine

In Greek sculpture there is a remarkable evolution from **rigid young men** (Fig. 66) standing up symmetrically (inherited from the Egyptians) to **the Apollo of Praxiteles** (Fig. 67), whose fluidity gives more life to marble or bronze. This sculptor of genius invented the **praxitelian position**, the asymmetrical position of one-legged standing, which has since inspired the entire art of sculpture. Long before our military the Greek sculptors had already invented the positions of standing at attention and standing at ease!

This praxitelian position is adopted in numerous activities of daily life, particularly among artisans and musicians. For **violinists** (Fig. 68) the pelvis is symmetrical most of the time, but the shoulder girdle must take up a very asymmetrical position, driving the cervical spine into a very abnormal stance. Thus these artists often have problems that may have a serious impact on their careers and may require the help of highly specialized experts in rehabilitation.

All stringed instruments necessitate an asymmetrical posture. In **guitarists** (Fig. 69) there is asymmetry not only of the shoulder girdle but also of the pelvis, as the left foot is raised on a wedge. **Pianists** need to rest their pelves properly, and for a pianist the adjustment of the seat is of great importance:

- if the seat is **at the right distance and at the right height** (Fig. 70) the spinal curvatures are normal and the shoulder girdle is so positioned that the upper limbs can reach the keyboard *without effort or contortion*
- if the seat is **too far back** (Fig. 71) the spine assumes an abnormal position and *both the thoracic and lumbar curvatures are exaggerated* to allow the hands to reach the keyboard. Moreover, the *shoulder girdle tires easily* because of the excessive distance between hands and seat.

Even when the seat is properly adjusted, pianists must know how to control their lumbar spines (Fig. 72), since lumbago can result from constant lumbar hyperlordosis.

To summarize, it is easy to see that it is of fundamental importance for **musicians**, especially those **who play string instruments, to exercise proper control over their spines at rest.** In fact, the quality of their work and artistry can suffer from **longstanding poor posture**, which is often difficult to correct even by prolonged rehabilitation under the care of **specialized physiotherapists.** The spine plays a crucial role in supporting the **shoulder girdle**, which often functions in **asymmetrical positions**, so that *longstanding bad posture can have disastrous consequences*. Musicians must therefore *take great care of their spines.*

Fig. 66

Fig. 67

Fig. 68

Fig. 69

Fig. 70

Fig. 71

Fig. 72

125

The spine in the sitting and recumbent positions

Sitting positions

In the sitting position with ischial support (Fig. 73), as when *a typist* is typing without resting her back on a chair, the full weight of the trunk is borne only by the ischia, while the pelvis is in a state of unstable equilibrium and tends to tilt forward, thereby increasing all three vertebral curvatures. The muscles of the shoulder girdle – especially the trapezius which slings the shoulder girdle and the upper limbs – are recruited to stabilize the spine. In the long run this position causes **the painful condition of the typist's syndrome or the trapezius syndrome.**

In the sitting position with ischiofemoral support (Fig. 74), as that of the *coachman*, the flexed trunk, even when it is occasionally propped up on the knees by the arms, is supported by the *ischial tuberosities and the posterior surfaces of the thighs.* The pelvis is tilted forward, the thoracic curvature is increased and the *lumbar curvature is straightened.* The arms stabilize the trunk with minimal muscular support and one can even fall asleep (as the coachman does). *This position rests the paravertebral muscles,* and is often adopted instinctively by **patients with spondylolisthesis**, since it *reduces the shearing forces on the lumbosacral disc* and *relaxes the posterior muscles.*

In the sitting position with ischiosacral support (Fig. 75) the whole trunk is *pulled back* so as to rest on the back of a chair and is supported by the *ischial tuberosities* and the *posterior surfaces of the sacrum and coccyx.* **The pelvis is now tilted backwards, the lumbar curvature is flattened**, the thoracic curvature is increased and the head can bend forward on the thorax, while the cervical curvature is inverted. This is also a **position of rest**, where *sleep is possible* but *breathing is hampered* by the neck flexion and the weight of the head resting on the sternum. This position *reduces the anterior slippage of L5* and relaxes the posterior lumbar muscles **with relief of the pain caused by spondylolisthesis.**

The recumbent positions

The supine position with lower limbs extended (Fig. 76) is the one most often adopted for resting. The psoas major muscles are stretched and the lumbar hyperlordosis hollows the loins.

In the supine position with lower limbs flexed (Fig. 77) the **psoas muscles are relaxed**, the *pelvis is tilted backwards* and the **lumbar curvature is flattened.** As a result, the **loins** rest directly on the supporting surface with even better relaxation of the spinal and abdominal muscles.

In the so-called position of relaxation (Fig. 78), secured with the help of cushions or specially designed chairs, the supporting thoracic region is concave, resulting in the flattening of the lumbar and cervical curvatures. **If the knees are supported**, the hips are flexed and the psoas major and hamstrings muscles are relaxed.

During side-lying (Fig. 79) the spine becomes *sinuous* and the lumbar curvature convex. The line joining the sacral fossae and the line joining the shoulders converge at a point above the subject. The thoracic spine becomes convex superiorly. This position *cannot relax the muscles in general* and *causes some respiratory difficulties during anaesthesia.*

The prone position is bedevilled by the adverse effects of an exaggerated lumbar curvature and respiratory difficulties. These difficulties are due to pressure on the thoracic cage, displacement of the abdominal viscera towards the diaphragm, reduction of its excursion and possible obstruction of the carina by external pressure, secretions and foreign bodies. Nevertheless, many people adopt this position to fall asleep but change position during sleep. In general, *a single position is never kept for long during sleep*, and this is to allow **all muscle groups to relax in succession**, and above all to **rotate the pressure areas.** It is well known that **when pressure areas are maintained for over 3 hours, ischaemic pressure or patches of skin necrosis of variable depth sores will develop.**

Fig. 73

Fig. 74

Fig. 76

Fig. 75

Fig. 77

Fig. 78

Fig. 79

127

Range of flexion-extension of the lumbar spine

The range of these movements varies with the subject and with age. All the values given will therefore be particular cases or averages (Fig. 80):

- **extension** associated with *lumbar hyperlordosis* has a range of 30°.
- **flexion** associated with *straightening of the lumbar curvature* has a range of 40°.

The work of David Allbrook (Fig. 81) allows us to know the individual ranges of flexion-extension at every spinal level (right column) and the total cumulative range (left column), which is 83° (i.e. close to the 70° value given previously).

On the other hand, **the range of flexion-extension is maximal between L4 and L5** (i.e. 24°), and it decreases progressively with values of 18° between L3 and L4 and L5 and S1, 12° between L2 and L3 and 11° between L1 and L2. Therefore, the *lower lumbar spine is considered to be more mobile in flexion-extension than the upper lumbar spine.*

As expected, the ranges of flexion vary with age (Fig. 82, inspired by Tanz). The mobility of the lumbar spine **decreases with age** and is maximal *between the ages of 2 and 13* Movement is greatest in the *lower part of the lumbar spine*, especially at level L4-L5.

Fig. 80

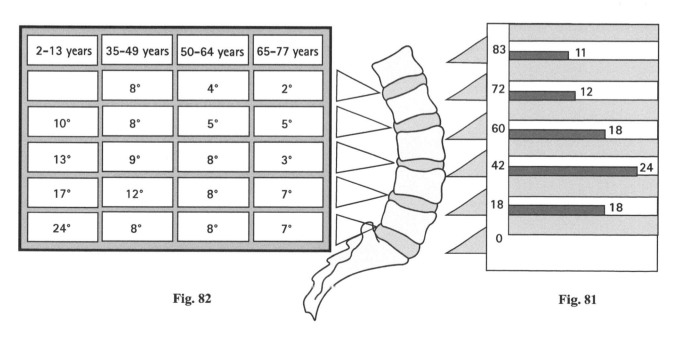

2–13 years	35–49 years	50–64 years	65–77 years
	8°	4°	2°
10°	8°	5°	5°
13°	9°	8°	3°
17°	12°	8°	7°
24°	8°	8°	7°

Fig. 82

Fig. 81

Range of lateral flexion of the lumbar spine

As with flexion-extension, the **range of lateral flexion** (Fig. 83) or inclination of the lumbar spine varies with the individual and with age. On average it can be said that lateral flexion on either side ranges from 20° to 30°.

Tanz (Fig. 84) has studied **the ranges of lateral flexion at each level of the spine**, and the global range decreases significantly with age:

- it is **maximal between 2 and 13 years of age**, when it reaches **62°** on either side of the midline
- between 35 and 49 years of age the range drops to 31°
- between 50 and 64 years it drops further to 29°
- between 65 and 77 years it reaches 22°.

Therefore, having remained maximal up to the age of 13, the global range of lateral flexion *remains relatively stable at about 30° from 35 to 64 years* and then drops to 20°. In middle age the full range of lateral flexion is **60°**, apparently equal to that of flexion-extension of the lumbar spine.

It is worth noting that the segmental range of lateral flexion at L5-S1 is very small as it rapidly drops from 7° in youth to 2° to 1° or even zero in old age. **It is maximal at L4–L5, and especially at L3–L4**, where it peaks at 16° in youth, stays relatively stable at 8° between 35 and 64 years and drops to 6° in old age.

Fig. 83

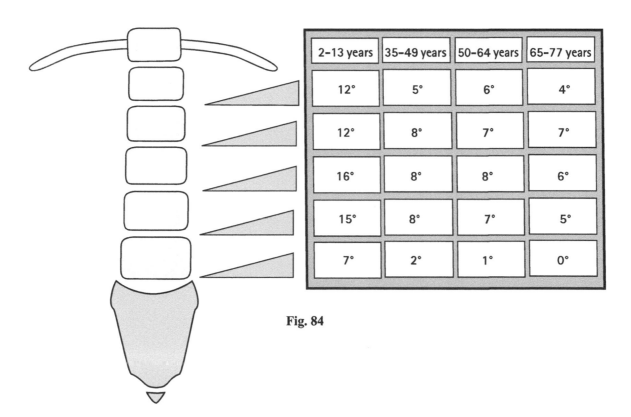

2–13 years	35–49 years	50–64 years	65–77 years
12°	5°	6°	4°
12°	8°	7°	7°
16°	8°	8°	6°
15°	8°	7°	5°
7°	2°	1°	0°

Fig. 84

Range of rotation of the thoracolumbar spine

The ranges of segmental and global rotation of the lumbar spine and of the thoracic spine have remained unknown for a long time. In fact, it is very difficult to fix the pelvis and measure the rotation of the thoracic spine, because the mobility of the scapular girdle on the thorax leaves a very wide margin of error. The recent work of Gregersen and Lucas has provided reliable measurements. These investigators did not hesitate *to implant under local anaesthesia metal pins* into the spinous processes of the thoracic and lumbar vertebrae in order to measure their angular displacements using *very sensitive recording devices*. They were thus able to measure the **rotation of the thoracolumbar spine during walking** (Fig. 85), **sitting and standing** (Fig. 86).

During walking (Fig. 85) the disc between T7 and T8 stays put (left curve L), while rotation is maximal at the discs immediately above and below (right part of diagram). It is therefore in the region of this **pivotal joint** that rotation has the greatest range, and then decreases progressively craniad and caudad to reach a minimum in the lumbar (0.3°) and in the upper thoracic (0.6°) segments, as shown by the curve R. **Thus rotation of the lumbar spine is only half of that present in the less mobile regions of the thoracic spine**; we have already seen the anatomical reasons for this limitation of movement.

In a study of the total and the maximal range of bilateral rotation (Fig. 87) Gregersen and Lucas show slight differences between the sitting (S) and the upright (U) positions. **In the sitting position** the values are smaller as the pelvis is more easily immobilized when the hips are flexed in order to define the reference coronal plane (C).

For the lumbar spine alone **the total range of bilateral rotation** is only 10°, i.e. 5° on either side and 1° on average at each vertebral level.

For the thoracic spine rotation is *appreciably greater*, amounting to 85° minus 10° or 75° bilaterally, **37° unilaterally and 34° on average unilaterally at each vertebral** level. Thus, *despite the presence of the thoracic cage*, global rotation is **four times greater in the thoracic spine** than in the lumbar spine. A comparison of the two curves (Fig. 86) reveals that both in the sitting and in the upright positions the total range of bilateral rotation is the same. There are only **segmental differences** between these two curves; for instance, the curve for the upright position (U) has four **points of inflexion**, with special emphasis on the points of inflexion **in the lowermost part of the lumbar spine, where rotation is maximal during standing**. The same applies to the transitional zone of the **thoracolumbar hinge**.

In practice, since it is impossible to implant metal pins into the spinous processes of subjects to study the rotation of the thoracolumbar spine, **old-fashioned clinical methods can be used in the sitting position** (Fig. 87) with the intershoulder line kept fixed relative to the thorax. The subject is then asked to rotate the trunk on one side and then the other, and the range of rotation is measured as the angle between the intershoulder line and the coronal plane (C). Here it is given as 15-20° but falls short of the 45° maximum given for unilateral rotation by Gregersen and Lucas. A practical way of stabilizing the scapular girdle relative to the thorax is to rest the upper arms horizontally on the *handle of a broom placed across the back at the level of the scapulae*. The broom handle then represents **the intershoulder line**.

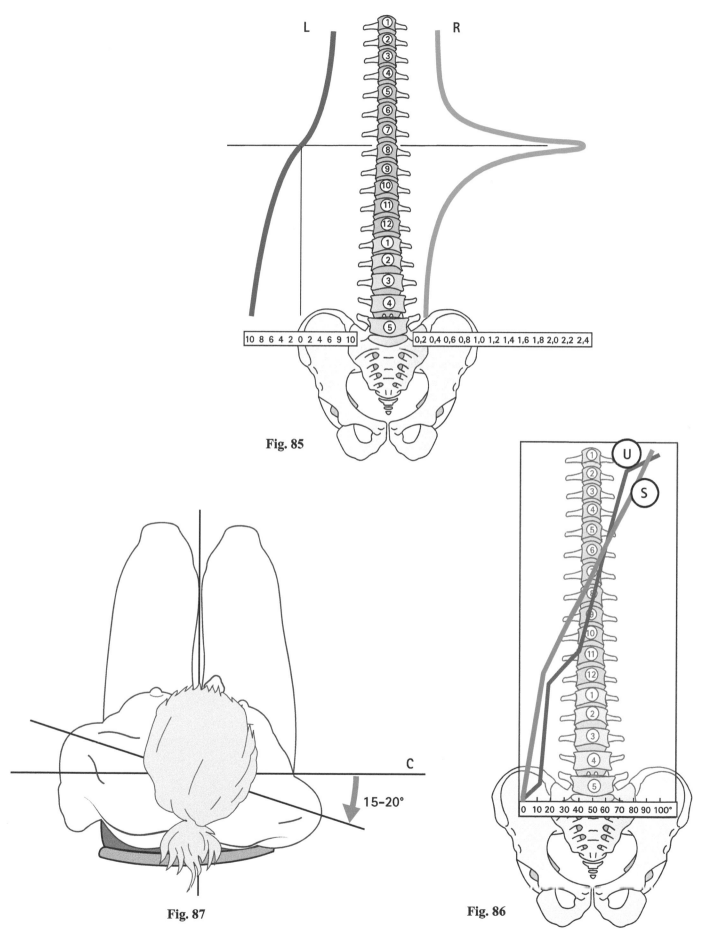

Fig. 85

Fig. 87

15-20°

Fig. 86

The intervertebral foramen and the radicular collar

It is impossible to close this chapter on the functional anatomy of the lumbar curve without some details of the physiopathology of the nerve roots, particularly prominent in this segment of the spine.

Some knowledge of anatomy is a prerequisite for understanding of nerve root lesions. **Each nerve root** (NR) exits the vertebral canal by an **intervertebral foramen** (2), which is bounded (Fig. 88) as follows:

- anteriorly, by the **posterior edge of the intervertebral disc** (1) and the adjacent parts of the vertebral bodies
- inferiorly, by the **pedicle of the underlying vertebra** (10)
- superiorly, by the **pedicle of the overlying vertebra** (11)
- posteriorly, by the **facet joints** (9) covered in front by their **capsule** (8) and the **lateral border of the ligamentum flavum** (6), which comes to lie on top of the capsule and *encroach slightly* on the intervertebral foramen, as shown in Figure 90.

Within the foramen (2) the nerve root must pierce the dura (Fig. 89); this lateral view in perspective shows how the **nerve root** (3) lies initially **within the dural sac** (14), approaches the internal aspect of the **dural sac** (4) and pierces it at the **radicular collar** (5). The nerve must pass through this fixed point, where it is *supported by the dural sac*.

In the spinal canal this dural sac corresponds to the **dura mater**, which is the outermost and strongest envelope of the nervous system.

Figure 90 (**superior view**) shows again all these relations between the neuraxis and the vertebral canal. The **spinal cord** (shown in cross-section) consists of **grey matter** centrally and of **white matter** peripherally; it is surrounded by the **dural sac** (4) and lies within the **vertebral canal**, which is covered as follows:

- anteriorly, by the **posterior longitudinal ligament** (12)
- posteriorly by the **ligamentum flavum** (7).

Anterior to the vertebral body the **longitudinal anterior ligament** (13) is seen in cross-section. The anterior aspect of the **facet joints** (9) is covered by a capsule and is reinforced by a **capsular ligament** (8) and by an **extension of the ligamentum flavum** (6). The **nerve root** (NR), resting on the **pedicle of the underlying vertebra** (10), passes through a **narrow tunnel** between:

- anteriorly, the intervertebral disc and the posterior longitudinal ligament
- posteriorly, the facet joint covered by an extension of the ligamentum flavum.

It is within the **confines of this intervertebral foramen**, bounded by solid and thus inextensible components, that the nerve root can be threatened and compressed by a **prolapsed disc.**

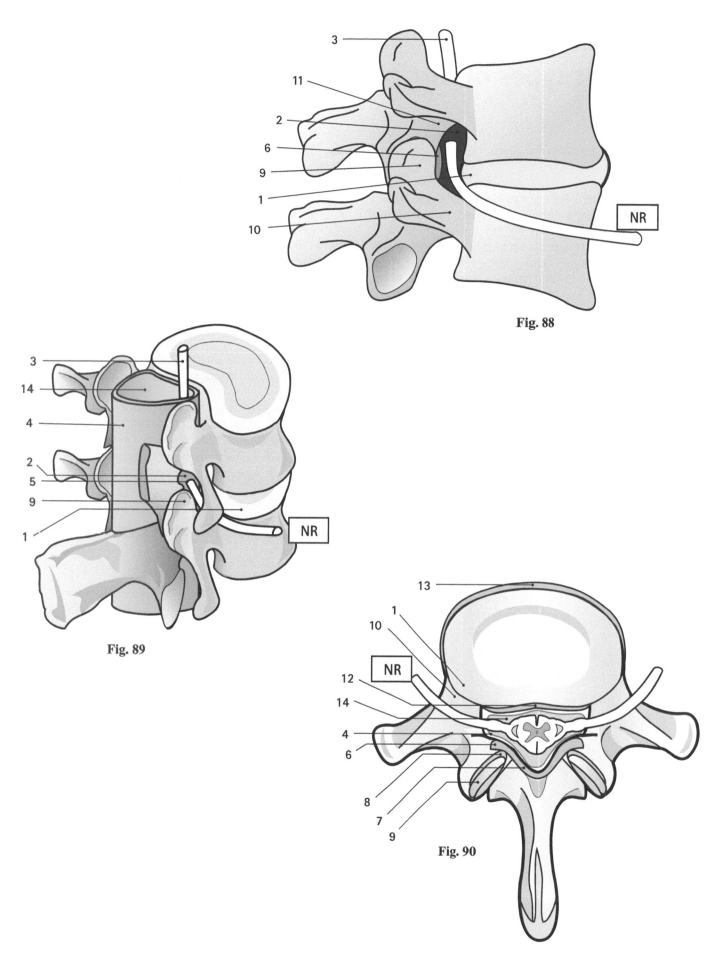

Fig. 88

Fig. 89

Fig. 90

The legends are the same for all figures.

135

The various types of disc prolapse

When compressed axially, the substance of the nucleus pulposus can stream out in various directions.

If the fibres of the annulus fibrosus are still strong enough, the increased pressure within the nucleus can cause the **vertebral discal surfaces to give way**. This corresponds to **intravertebral prolapse** (Fig. 91).

Recent studies have shown that the annulus fibres start to degenerate after 25 years of age, leading to tears within its various bundles. Therefore, under axial stresses, the **nuclear material can stream out through the torn fibres of the annulus** (Fig. 92) in a **concentric** or more often **radial** fashion. The prolapse of nuclear material anteriorly is among the rarest, whereas posterior prolapse and particularly **posterolateral prolapse** are almost the rule.

Therefore, when the **disc is crushed** (Fig. 93), part of the nuclear substance escapes anteriorly, but more likely posteriorly and can thus reach the posterior edge of the disc to emerge under the **posterior longitudinal ligament** (Fig. 94).

After the annulus is split (A), a streamer from the nucleus, still attached to it, can remain trapped under the posterior longitudinal ligament (B), whence it can be brought back by vertebral traction produced by stretching the trunk, but more often it **snaps the posterior longitudinal ligament** (C) and may even come to **lie free within the vertebral canal**, i.e. the **free or migrating type of disc prolapse** (D). In other cases, the nuclear streamer **stays trapped under the posterior longitudinal ligament** (E) and gets nipped off by the fibres of the annulus, which snap back into position and preclude any return to normal.

Finally, in other cases the streamer reaches the deep surface of the posterior longitudinal ligament and glides inferiorly or superiorly (F). This corresponds to the migrating subligamentous prolapse.

It is only when the prolapsed disc presses against the deep surface of the posterior longitudinal ligament that nerve endings within the ligament are stretched causing **lumbago** or a sprained back.

Finally, compression of the nerve root by the prolapsed disc causes **nerve root pain**, which has different names according to its location. For example, it is called **sciatica** when the sciatic nerve is involved. The term **lumbago-sciatica** is often used since at the start the sciatica is associated with low back pain.

Fig. 91

Fig. 92

Fig. 93

A

B

C

D

E

F

Fig. 94

Disc prolapse and the mechanism of nerve root compression

It is now generally accepted that **disc prolapse occurs in three stages**, but it only occurs if the disc has previously *deteriorated as a result of repeated microtraumas* and if the annulus fibres have started *to degenerate*.

Disc prolapse usually follows the **lifting of a weight** with the trunk *flexed forward*.

- **During the first stage** (Fig. 95) trunk flexion flattens the disc anteriorly and *widens* the intervertebral space *posteriorly*. The nuclear material is *driven posteriorly* through the pre-existing tears in the annulus.
- **During the second stage** (Fig. 96), as soon as the weight is lifted, the increased axial compression crushes the whole disc and **violently drives the nuclear material posteriorly** until it reaches the deep surface of the posterior longitudinal ligament.
- **During the third stage** (Fig. 97), when the trunk is nearly straight, the zigzagging path taken by the pedicle of the herniating mass is closed by the pressure of the vertebral discal surfaces, and the herniated mass stays trapped under the posterior longitudinal ligament. This causes the **violent acute pain** in the loin or **lumbago**, which is the **initial phase of the lumbago-sciatica complex.**

This initial acute lumbago *can regress spontaneously* or *with treatment*, but as a result of similar repeated traumas, the hernia *grows in size* and protrudes more and more into the vertebral canal. At this point it **comes into contact with one of the nerve roots**, often that of the sciatic nerve (Fig. 98).

The hernia usually starts at the **posterolateral part of the disc**, where the posterior longitudinal ligament is at its thinnest, and progressively pushes the sciatic nerve root along until its excursion is stopped by the *posterior wall of the intervertebral foramen*, i.e. *the facet joint reinforced by its capsule, its anterior capsular ligament and the lateral border of the ligamentum flavum*. From now on, the compression-damaged nerve root will give rise to pain felt in **its corresponding body segment** and eventually to impaired reflexes (e.g. *the loss of Achilles' tendon reflex* **when S1 is compressed**) and to **motor disturbances** as **in sciatica-associated paralysis.**

The clinical picture (Fig. 99) depends on the spinal level of disc prolapse and nerve root compression.

- When the prolapse occurs at L4-L5 (1), the root of L5 is compressed and pain is felt in **the posterolateral aspect of the thigh and of the knee, the lateral border of the calf, the dorsolateral border of the instep and the dorsal surface of the foot down to the big toe.**
- When the prolapse occurs at L5-S1 (2), S1 is compressed and the pain is referred to the **posterior surface of the thigh, knee and calf, the heel and the lateral border of the foot down to the little toe.** It can be associated with loss of the Achilles tendon reflex.

This generalization needs to be qualified, since a hernia at L4-L5 may lie closer to the midline and **compress both L5 and S1** or even **occasionally S1 only.** Surgical exploration of the L5-S1 interspace, performed on the basis of the S1 root pain, *may fail to recognize the lesion that lies one level above*.

The **sagittal section** (Fig. 99) shows that in fact **the spinal cord stops at L2 to become the conus medullaris** (CM). Below the conus the dural sac contains only the nerve roots gathered **in the cauda equina**, and they emerge two by two at each level through the intervertebral foramina. The dural sac ends in a cul-de-sac (D) at the level of S3. The lumbar plexus (LP), made up of L3-L5, gives rise to the **femoral nerve** (F). The sacral plexus (SP), consisting of the **lumbosacral trunk** (LS), i.e. branch of L4 + L5 + S1-S3, gives rise to the two branches of the sciatic nerve (S), i.e. the common peroneal and the tibial nerves.

Fig. 95

Fig. 96

Fig. 97

Fig. 99

Fig. 98

Lasègue's sign

Lasègue's sign is the **pain induced by stretching the sciatic nerve or one of its roots.** It is elicited by *gradual and slow elevation of the extended lower limb* with *the patient supine.* The pain induced is similar to that felt spontaneously by the patient, i.e. *in the same topographic distribution as the affected nerve root.* Charnley has shown that **the nerve roots glide freely through the intervertebral foramina** and that, during elevation of the lower limb with the knee extended, **the nerve roots are pulled out of the intervertebral foramina** for a distance of **12 mm** at the level of L5 (Fig. 100).

Lasègue's sign can therefore be interpreted as follows:
- When the subject is **supine with the lower limbs resting on a supporting surface** (Fig. 101) the sciatic nerve and its roots are *under no tension at all.*
- When the **lower limb is elevated with the knee flexed** (Fig. 102) the sciatic nerve and its roots are *still under no tension.*
- But if the knee is then extended or if **the lower limb is progressively elevated with the knee extended** (Fig. 103), the sciatic nerve, which must now run a longer course, is subjected *to increasing tension.*

In the normal subject the *nerve roots glide freely through the intervertebral foramina* and this procedure elicits no pain at all; only when the limb is almost vertical (Fig. 104) is **pain felt on the posterior aspect of the thigh** as a result of **stretching of the hamstrings** in people with reduced flexibility. This is a *false-positive Lasègue sign.*

Obviously when one of the roots is trapped in the intervertebral foramen or when it must run a slightly longer course over the bulge of a prolapsed disc, any stretching of the nerve will become painful **even with moderate elevation of the lower limb.** This is a **true-positive Lasègue sign**, which is generally evident before 60° of flexion is attained. In fact, after 60°, the Lasègue sign is not applicable, since the sciatic nerve is already **maximally stretched at 60°.** Thus pain may be elicited at 10°, 15° or 20° elevation of the lower limb and the test **can be quantified as positive** at 10°, 15°, 20° or 30°.

One point needs to be stressed. During forced elevation of the limb with the knee extended the **force of traction on the nerve roots is 3 kg**, whereas the resistance of these roots to traction is 3.2 kg. Therefore, if a root is trapped or relatively shortened by a herniated disc, **any rough manipulation can rupture some axons within the nerve root**, resulting in some form of **paralysis**, which is usually short-lived but occasionally *may take a long time to subside.* Therefore, **two precautions must be taken:**
- The test must be carried out **gently and cautiously** and *must be stopped as soon as the patient feels any pain.*
- **It must never be performed under general anaesthesia**, since the protective effect of pain is lost. This can occur when the patient **is being placed in the prone position on the operating table** for a herniated disc repair and the hips are flexed while the **knees remain extended.** The surgeon must always **personally place the patient** on the table and make sure that **hip flexion is always associated with knee flexion**, which slackens the sciatic nerve and protects the trapped nerve root.

Fig. 101

Fig. 102

Fig. 103

Fig. 100

12 mm

Fig. 104

Chapter 4

THE THORACIC SPINE AND THE THORAX

The thoracic spine is the segment of the spine lying between the lumbar and cervical segments and forming the **axis of the upper part of the trunk.** It **supports the thorax**, which is a *cavity of variable capacity* bounded by 12 pairs of ribs articulating with the vertebrae. The thorax is committed to **respiration** and **houses the heart and the respiratory system.** The thoracic wall allows the thoracic spine to support the **shoulder girdle**, which articulates with the **upper limbs.**

Contrary to appearances, the thoracic spine is **more mobile in terms of rotation** than the lumbar spine. It is **far less affected by mechanical stresses**, and its lesions result essentially from acquired deformities.

The typical thoracic vertebra and the twelfth thoracic vertebra

The typical thoracic vertebra

This is made up of the same parts as the lumbar vertebra, with *important structural and functional differences.*

A 'disassembled' view (Fig. 1) shows the **vertebral body** (1) with roughly equal transverse and anteroposterior diameters. It is also *proportionately higher than the lumbar vertebra*, and its anterior and lateral surfaces are quite hollow.

The posterolateral corner of its superior surface bears an **oval articular** facet (13), obliquely set and lined by cartilage; this is the superior costal articular facet, which will be discussed later in relation to the costovertebral joints (see p. 151).

Posterolaterally the vertebral body bears **two pedicles** (2 and 3) and the superior costal facet often encroaches on the root of the pedicle.

Behind the pedicles arise the **laminae** (4 and 5), which form the bulk of the dorsal vertebral arches, are *higher than they are wide* and are arranged like *tiles on a roof.* Near the pedicles their superior borders give attachment to the **superior articular processes** (6 and 7), each fitted with an articular facet. These cartilage-coated facets are oval, flat or slightly convex transversely and face posteriorly and slightly superiorly and laterally. Near the pedicles their inferior borders give attachment to the **inferior articular processes** (only the **right process** is shown here as 8), which bear oval, flat or slightly transversely concave articular facets (7) facing anteriorly and slightly inferiorly and medially. Each inferior facet articulates with the superior facet of the upper vertebra at the **facet joint.**

The junction of the laminae and the pedicles at the level of the articular processes gives attachment to the **transverse processes** (9 and 11), facing laterally and slightly posteriorly. Their free extremities are bulbous and bear on their anterior surfaces small articular facets called the **transverse costal facets** (10), corresponding to the costal tubercles. These two laminae unite in the midline to form the long and bulky **spinous processes** (12), which are sharply inclined inferiorly and posteriorly and terminate as *single tubercles.*

All these components combine to form the **typical thoracic vertebra** (Fig. 2). In the diagram, the two red arrows indicate the posterior, lateral and slightly superior orientation of the articular facets of the superior articular processes.

The twelfth thoracic vertebra (T12)

The **last thoracic vertebra** (T12) acts as a bridge between the thoracic and lumbar regions (Fig. 3) and has some characteristics of its own:

- Its body has only **two costal facets**, located at the posterolateral angles of its *superior surface* and destined for the *heads of the twelfth ribs.*
- Whereas its superior articular processes are oriented (red arrows) like those of the other thoracic vertebrae (i.e. posteriorly, slightly superiorly and laterally), its inferior articular processes must conform to those of L1. Therefore, like all of the lumbar vertebrae (blue arrow), they face *laterally and anteriorly* and are slightly convex transversely as they describe in space *similar cylindrical surfaces* with centres of curvature lying roughly at the *base of each spinous process.*

Fig. 1

Fig. 2

Fig. 3

145

Flexion-extension and lateral flexion of the thoracic spine

During extension between two thoracic vertebrae (Fig. 4) the upper vertebra tilts posteriorly relative to the lower vertebra, and the intervertebral disc is *flattened posteriorly and widened anteriorly* while the nucleus pulposus is driven *anteriorly*, as is the case with the lumbar vertebrae. Extension is limited by the **impact of the articular processes** (1) **and of the spinous processes** (2), which are sharply bent inferiorly and posteriorly and are already almost in contact with one another. Furthermore, the **anterior longitudinal ligament** (3) is stretched, while the **posterior longitudinal ligament, the ligamenta flava and the interspinous ligaments** are slackened.

Conversely, **during flexion between two thoracic vertebrae** (Fig. 5), the *intervertebral space gapes posteriorly*, and the nucleus is displaced *posteriorly*. The articular surfaces of the articular processes glide **upwards**, and the inferior articular processes of the overlying vertebra tend to **overshoot from above** the superior processes of the underlying vertebra. Flexion is limited by the tension developed in the **interspinous ligaments** (4), the **ligamenta flava**, the **capsular ligaments of the facet joints** (5) and the **posterior longitudinal ligaments** (6). On the other hand, *the anterior longitudinal ligament is slackened*.

During lateral flexion between two thoracic vertebrae (Fig. 6, posterior view), the articular facets of the facet joints **glide relative to one another** as follows:

- on the contralateral side, the facets glide as they do during flexion, i.e. upwards (red arrow)
- on the ipsilateral side, the facets glide as they do during extension, i.e. downwards (blue arrow).

The line joining the two transverse processes of the upper vertebra (mm′) and the corresponding line for the lower vertebra (nn′) form an **angle equal to that of lateral flexion** (lf).

Lateral flexion is limited:

- ipsilaterally by the **impact of the articular processes**
- contralaterally by the **stretching of the ligamenta flava and of the intertransverse ligaments**.

It would be incorrect to consider the movements of the thoracic spine only in terms of the individual vertebrae. In fact, the thoracic spine articulates with the thoracic cage or **thorax** (Fig. 7), and all the bony, cartilaginous and articular components of this bony cage play a role in orienting and limiting the isolated movements of the spine. Thus, in the cadaver, the isolated thoracic spine can be observed **to be more mobile** than the thoracic spine attached to the thoracic cage. Therefore, it is necessary to study **the changes in the thorax** induced by movements in the thoracic spine:

- **During lateral flexion of the thoracic spine** (Fig. 8) on the contralateral side the thorax is **elevated** (1), the intercostal spaces are **widened** (3), the thoracic cage is **enlarged** (5) and the **costochondral angle** of the tenth rib tends to **gape** (7). On the ipsilateral side, the opposite changes occur, i.e. the thorax moves **downwards** (2) **and inwards** (6), **the intercostal spaces are narrowed** (4) and the **costochondral angles close down** (8).
- **During flexion of the thoracic spine** (Fig. 9) all the angles widen between the various segments of the thorax and between the thorax and the thoracic spine, i.e. the **costovertebral angle** (1), the **superior** (2) and **inferior** (3) **sternocostal angles** and the **costochondral angle** (4). Conversely, during extension *all these angles close down*.

Fig. 4

Fig. 5

Fig. 6

Fig. 7

Fig. 8

Fig. 9

147

Axial rotation of the thoracic spine

The mechanism of axial rotation of one thoracic vertebra over another differs from that of a lumbar vertebra. **When viewed from above** (Fig. 10) the facet joints have a totally different orientation. The profile of each joint space also describes a *cylindrical surface* (dotted circle), but the axis of this cylinder runs more or less **through the centre of the vertebral body** (O). When one vertebra rotates on another the articular facets of the articular processes glide one on the other and the vertebral bodies rotate relative to each other around their common axis. This is followed by **rotation-torsion** of the **intervertebral disc** and *not by shearing movements of the disc*, as in the lumbar region. The range of this rotation-torsion of the disc can be greater than that of its shearing movements. Simple rotation of a thoracic vertebra on another is **at least three times greater** than that of a lumbar vertebra.

This rotation, however, would be even greater *if the thoracic spine were not so tightly connected to the bony thorax* that any movement at every level of the spine induces a similar movement in the **corresponding pair of ribs** (Fig. 11); however, this gliding movement of one pair of ribs on an underlying pair is limited by the **presence of the sternum**, which articulates with the ribs via the flexible *costal cartilages.*

Therefore, rotation of a vertebra will distort the corresponding rib pair **because of the elasticity of the ribs and especially of their cartilages.** These distortions include the following:

- **accentuation of the concavity of the rib on the side of rotation** (1)

- **flattening of the concavity of the rib on the opposite side** (2)
- **accentuation of the costochondral concavity on the side opposite to the rotation** (3)
- **flattening of the costochondral concavity on the side of rotation** (4).

During this movement, the **sternum is subject to shearing forces**, and it tends to assume a superoinferior obliquity in order to follow the rotation of the vertebral bodies. This induced obliquity of the sternum must be *quite small and virtually absent* as it cannot be detected clinically; it is also difficult to detect radiologically because of the superimposition of multiple planes. *The mechanical resistance of the thorax therefore plays a role in appreciably limiting the range of motion of the thoracic spine.* When the thorax is still flexible, as in *the young*, movements of the thoracic spine have a sizable range, but in *the elderly the costal cartilages ossify* with a drop in costochondral elasticity, and the thorax **forms an almost rigid structure with decreased mobility.**

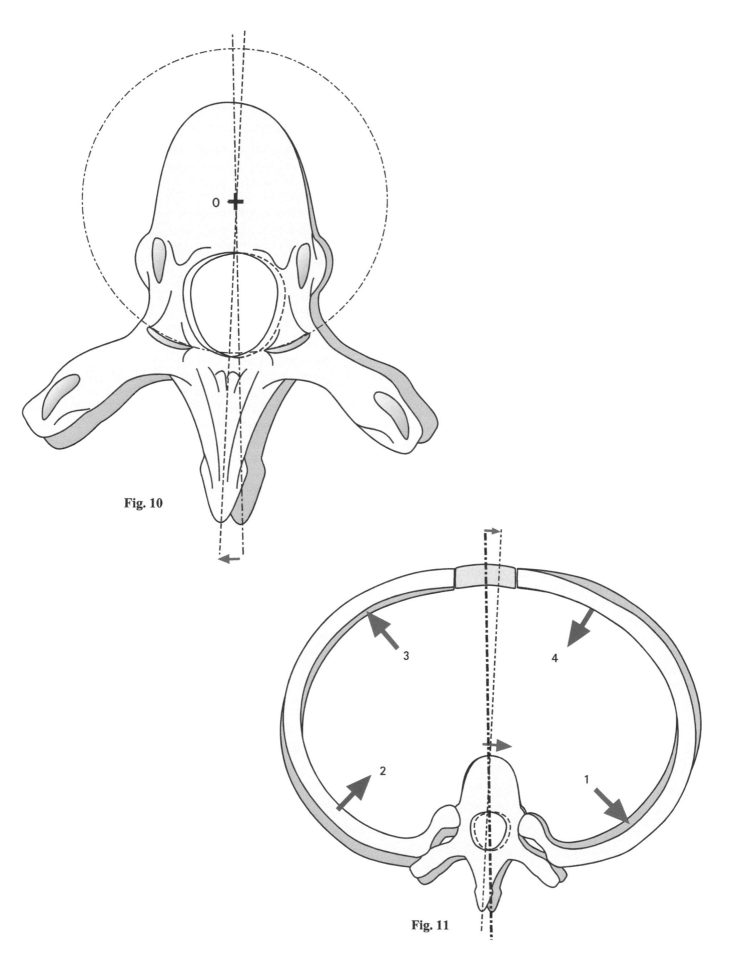

Fig. 10

Fig. 11

The costovertebral joints

At every level of the thoracic spine a pair of ribs articulates with the vertebra by means of **two costovertebral joints:**
- the **joint of costal head** (articulatio capitis costae) between the *head of the rib* and the *bodies of two adjacent vertebrae* and the *intervertebral disc*
- the **costotransverse joint** (articulatio costotransversaria) between the *costal tubercle* and the *transverse process* of the underlying vertebra.

Figure 12 (**side view**) shows one rib removed and some ligaments resected so as to reveal the vertebral articular facets; the underlying rib is left in place with its ligaments.

Figure 13 (**superior view**) shows the right rib in position but the joints have been opened; the left rib has been removed after resection of the ligaments.

Figure 14 (**verticofrontal view**) passes through the joint between the costal head and the vertebral bodies; on the other side, the rib has been removed after resection of the ligaments.

The **joint of costal head** is a double *synovial joint* made up on the vertebral side of **two costal facets**, one on the *superior border* of the lower vertebra (5) and the other on the *inferior border* of the upper vertebra (6). These facets form a *solid angle* (shown as red dashed lines in Fig. 14), whose *base* consists of the annulus fibrosus (2) of the *intervertebral disc*. The slightly convex corresponding facets (11 and 12) on the **head of the rib** (10) also form a solid angle, which *fits snugly* into the angle between the vertebral facets.

An **interosseous ligament** (8), running from the apex of the costal head between the two articular facets to the *intervertebral disc*, divides this joint, surrounded by a **single capsule** (9), into *two distinct joint cavities*, superior and inferior (13).

This joint is reinforced by a **radiate ligament** consisting of three bands:
- a **superior band** (14) and an **inferior band** (15), both inserted into the adjacent vertebrae

- an **intermediate band** (16) inserted into the **annulus fibrosus** (2) of the intervertebral disc.

The **costotransverse joint** is also a synovial joint consisting of *two oval articular facets*, one on the **apex of the transverse process** (18) and the other on the **costal tubercle** (19). It is surrounded by a single **capsule** (20), but it is reinforced above all by **three costotransverse ligaments:**
- the **very short and very strong interosseous costotransverse ligament** (23), running from the transverse process to the posterior aspect of the neck of the rib
- the **posterior costotransverse ligament** (21), rectangular in shape and 1.5 cm long and 1 cm wide; it runs from the apex of the transverse process (22) to the external border of the costal tubercle
- the **superior costotransverse ligament** (24), very thick and very strong, flat and quadrilateral, 8 mm wide and 10 mm long; it runs from the inferior border of the transverse process to the superior border of the neck of the underlying rib.

Some authors also describe an **inferior costotransverse ligament** lying on the inferior surface of the joint (not shown here). These diagrams also show the intervertebral disc with its **nucleus pulposus** (1) and its **annulus fibrosus** (2), the **vertebral canal** (C), the **intervertebral foramen** (F), the **vertebral pedicle** (P), the **facet joints** with their **articular facets** (3) and **their capsules** (4) and the **spinous processes** (7).

In summary, the rib articulates with the spine via two synovial joints:
- a **single joint**, the costotransverse joint
- a **double, more solidly interlocked joint**, the joint of costal head.

These two joints are supplied by powerful ligaments and cannot function one without the other (i.e. they are **mechanically linked**).

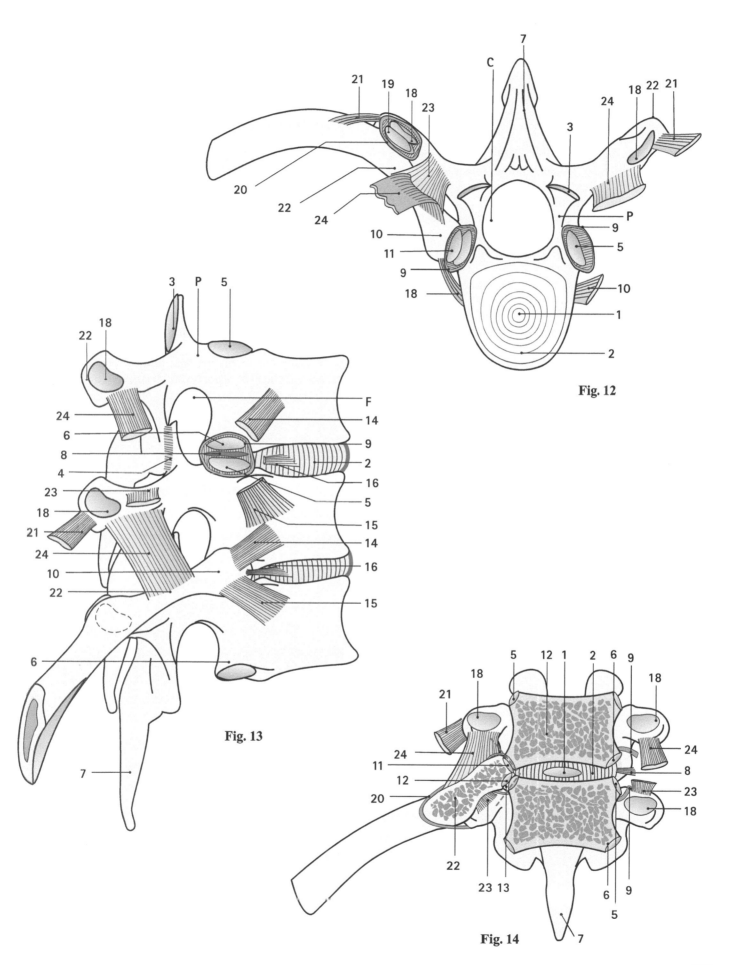

Fig. 12

Fig. 13

Fig. 14

151

The legends are the same for all figures.

Rib movements at the joints of costal heads

The joint of costal head and the costotransverse joint form a **couple of mechanically linked synovial joints** (Fig. 15) which share only one movement, i.e. **rotation** about a common axis passing through the centre of each joint.

This axis **xx′**, joining the centre **o′** of the costotransverse joint to the centre **o** of the joint of costal head, acts as a **swivel** for the rib, which is thus **literally 'suspended'** from the spine at two points **o** and **o′**.

The orientation of this axis relative to the sagittal plane *determines the direction of movement* of the rib. For the **lower ribs** (left side, lower) the axis **xx′** *moves closer to the sagittal plane* so that elevation of the rib **increases the transverse diameter** of the thorax by a length **t**. Thus, when the rib rotates about this axis **o′** (Fig. 16), its lateral border describes an arc of a circle with centre **o′**: it becomes less oblique and *more transverse,* and as a result its most lateral border moves **outwards** over a length **t**, which represents the **increase in the transverse hemidiameter** of the base of the thorax.

On the other hand, the axis **yy′** for the **upper ribs** (Fig. 15, right side, upper) lies almost in the *coronal plane.* Therefore, elevation of these ribs **markedly increases the anteroposterior diameter** of the thorax by a distance **a**. In effect, when the **anterior extremity of the rib rises by a distance h**, it describes an arc of a circle and is displaced anteriorly by a **length a** (Fig. 17).

It follows therefore that rib elevation **increases simultaneously the transverse diameter of the lower thorax and the anteroposterior diameter of the upper thorax.** In the midthoracic region, the joints of costal heads have an axis **running obliquely at roughly 45° to the sagittal plane so that both the transverse and the anteroposterior diameters are increased.**

Fig. 15

Fig. 16

Fig. 17

153

Movements of the costal cartilages and of the sternum

So far only the movements of the ribs at the costovertebral joints have been considered, but **their movements relative to the sternum and costal cartilages** also deserve attention. From a comparison of a **superior view** (Fig. 18) and of an **inferior view** (Fig. 19) of these rib movements, it is clear that, whereas the most lateral part of the rib **rises by a height of h′** and moves away from the axis of symmetry of the body by a length t′, the anterior end of the rib rises by a **height of h** and moves away from the axis of symmetry of the body by a length t. (Note that **h′** is slightly greater than **h**, since the most lateral part of the rib is farther removed from the centre of rotation than its anterior end.) At the same time, the sternum rises and the **costal cartilage becomes more horizontal**, forming an **angle (a)** with its initial position.

This angular movement of the costal cartilage relative to the sternum occurs at the **costosternal joint**; at the same time, there is another movement of angular rotation around the axis of the cartilage taking place at the costochondral joint. This will be discussed later (see p. 179).

During rib elevation (Fig. 18, right side) the point **m**, corresponding to the point of maximum increase in the thoracic diameter, is also the point most distant from the axis **yy′**. This geometrical observation explains how the degree of displacement of this point varies from rib to rib with the obliquity of their axes (xx′).

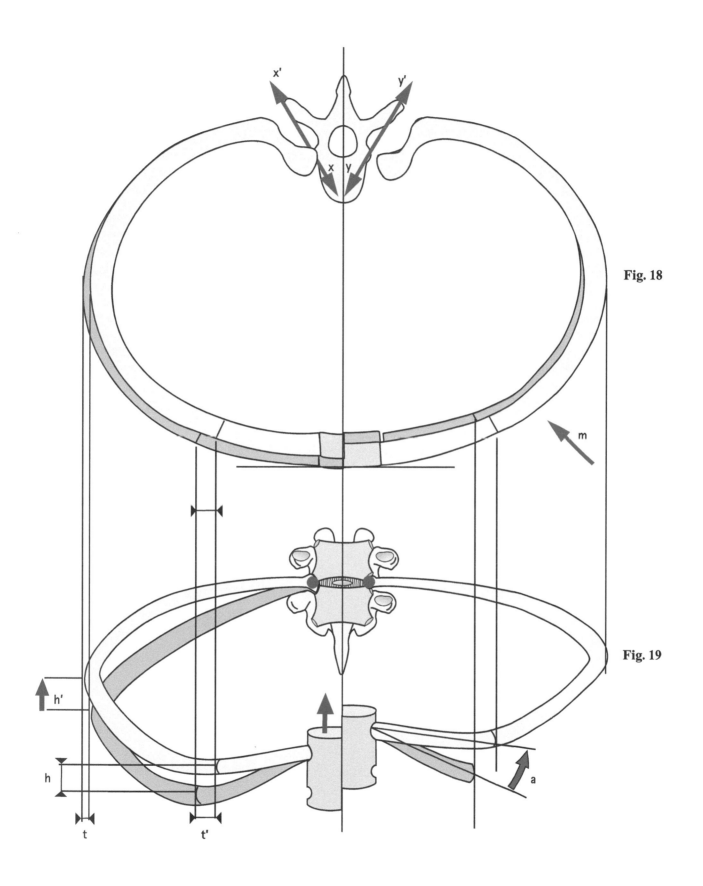

Fig. 18

Fig. 19

The deformations of the thorax in the sagittal plane during inspiration

Supposing that the spine remains fixed during inspiration without any deformation, one need only consider the changes in shape of the **flexible irregular pentagon** formed, on the one hand, by the **spine** (Fig. 20) and, on the other, by the *first rib, the sternum, the tenth rib and its costal cartilage.* The changes during inspiration are as follows:

- The **first rib**, being freely mobile at its joint of costal head (O), is **elevated** (blue arrow), so that its anterior extremity describes an **arc of a circle AA'**.
- As the first rib is elevated, **so is the sternum**, which **moves from AB to AB'**.
- During this movement, *the sternum does not stay parallel to itself.* As we have already seen, the anteroposterior diameter of the upper thorax is increased more than that of the lower thorax; it follows that the **angle (a)** between the sternum and the vertical plane **becomes slightly narrower** as does angle **OA'B'** *between the first rib and the sternum.*

This closure of the sternocostal angle is by necessity associated with **torsion of the costal cartilage** (see p. 179).

- The **tenth rib** is also raised *with Q as its centre of rotation,* while its anterior extremity describes an **arc of a circle CC'**.
- Finally, as both the tenth rib and the sternum are elevated, **the tenth costal cartilage moves from CB to C'B'** while staying roughly parallel to itself. It follows that during this movement the angle at **C** becomes greater at **C'** by a value of **c**, which is itself equal to the angle of elevation of the tenth rib (green triangles). At the same time, the angle between the tenth costal cartilage and the sternum (the angle **C'B'A'**) is slightly widened as a result once more of **torsion** of the cartilage on its long axis. **A similar degree of torsion occurs at every costal cartilage.** We shall see later its relevance as regards the elasticity of the thorax (see p. 179).

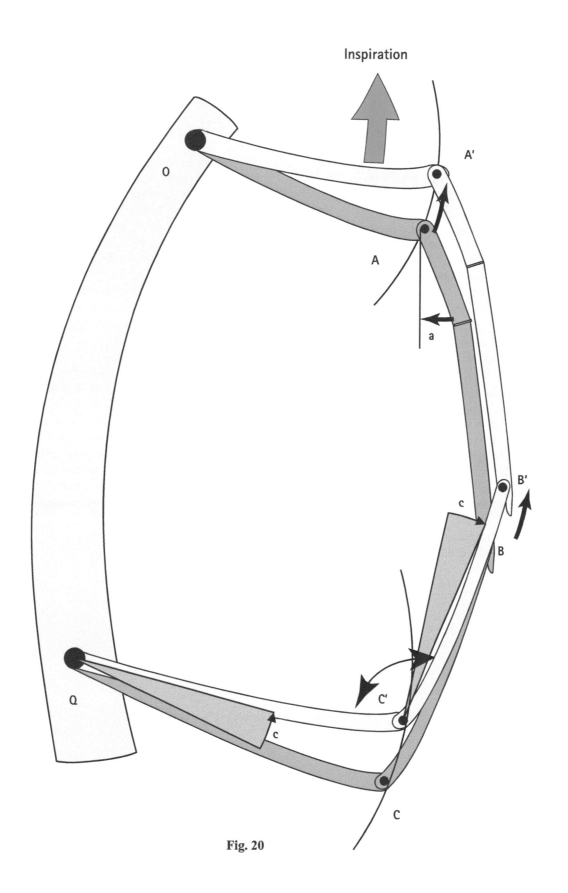

Fig. 20

Mode of action of the intercostal and sternocostal muscles

The intercostal muscles

A posterior view of the thorax, featuring only the spine and three ribs on the right side (Fig. 21), reveals the presence of **three muscles:**

- The small **levator costae muscles** (LC) stretch from the tip of the transverse process to the upper border of the rib below. Their contraction elevates the ribs; hence their name.

- The **external intercostal muscles** (E) run *obliquely, superiorly and medially parallel to those of the levator costae.* Therefore these muscles and the levator costae *elevate the rib* and act as **inspiratory** muscles.

- The **internal intercostal muscles** (I) run obliquely, superiorly and laterally. They depress the ribs and so are **expiratory** muscles.

The **mode of action of these intercostal muscles** is well explained by **Hamberger's diagram** (Figs 22 and 23):

- The action of the **external intercostals** (Fig. 22) is easily understood by the fact that the direction of their fibres is the same as that of the **long diagonal of the parallelogram $OO'B_1A_1$**, formed by the ribs articulating with the spine and the sternum. When the muscle **E** contracts, the shortening of this diagonal by a length **r** distorts the parallelogram and causes A_1 to rotate to A_2 and B_1 to B_2, assuming that OO' stays put. Therefore, since its contraction elevates the rib, the external intercostal is an **inspiratory muscle.**

- The action of the **internal intercostals** (Fig. 23) can be understood in the same way, but this time the direction of their fibres is parallel to the short diagonal of the parallelogram. When the muscle (I) contracts, the shortening of this diagonal $O'A_1$ by a length **r'** causes A_1 to rotate to A_2 and B_1 to B_2, still assuming that the side OO' stays put. Thus, since its contraction depresses the rib, it is an **expiratory muscle.**

Hamberger's demonstration was at one time contradicted by Duchenne de Boulogne's electrical stimulation experiments, but it is **now validated** by electromyographic studies.

The sternocostalis

The **sternocostalis** has received little study and tends to be ignored because of its **retrosternal location** (Fig. 24). It lies entirely on the *deep surface of the sternum* and its fibres, inserted into the cartilages of the second to sixth ribs, run *an oblique course inferiorly and medially.* Contraction of its five bundles depresses the corresponding costal cartilages *relative to the sternum.* We have already seen (Fig. 19, p. 155) that the costal cartilage is raised during inspiration and depressed during expiration. Therefore we can deduce that **the sternocostalis is an expiratory muscle.**

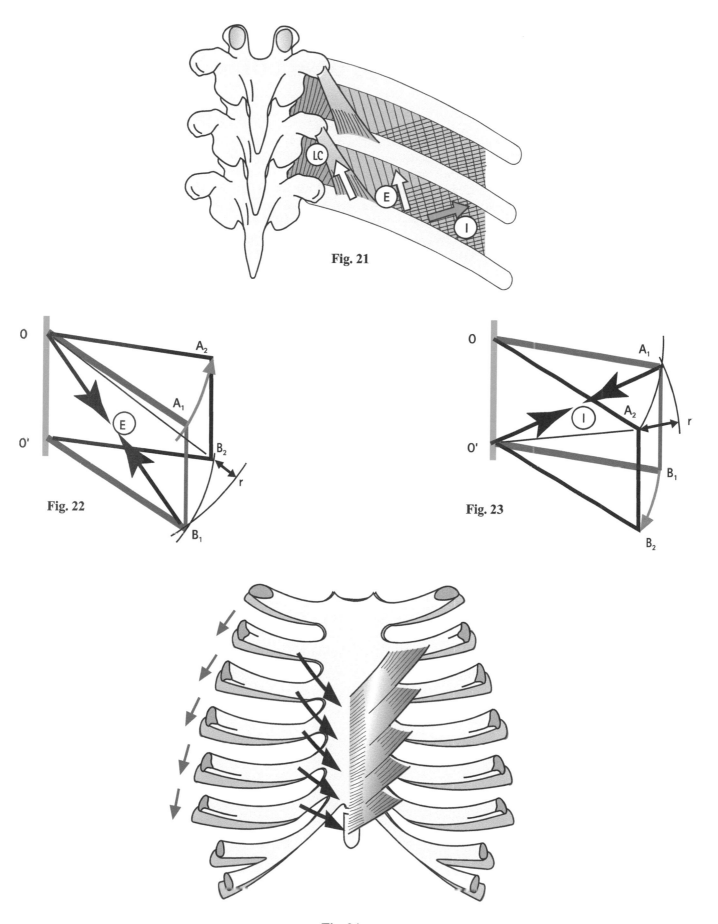

Fig. 21

Fig. 22

Fig. 23

Fig. 24

The diaphragm and its mode of action

The diaphragm is a **musculotendinous dome** closing the lower thoracic outlet and *separating the thorax from the abdomen.*

As seen from the side (Fig. 25) this dome reaches farther down posteriorly than anteriorly and its apex is the **central tendon** (1). From this central tendon **bundles of muscle fibres** (2) radiate out towards the rim of the thoracic outlet and are attached to the *deep surfaces of the costal cartilages,* the *tips of the eleventh and twelfth ribs,* the *costal arches* and finally the *vertebral bodies* by **two crura** as follows: the **left crus** (3) and the **right crus** (4) are attached respectively to the **medial arcuate ligament** (7) **arching over the psoas major and the lateral arcuate ligament** (8) **arching over the quadratus lumborum.**

This is more obvious **in the anterior view** (Fig. 26), where it is easy to recognize at the same time the *convex portion of the diaphragm* (the upper part of the diagram) and the *concave portion of the diaphragm* at the level of the crura. The **openings** in the diaphragm can also be seen as they allow the passage of the **oesophagus** (6) above and the **aorta** (5) below. For the sake of simplicity the opening for the inferior vena cava is not shown. When the diaphragm contracts the *central tendon is pulled down,* thereby *increasing the vertical diameter of the thorax.* Therefore, the diaphragm can be compared to a *piston* sliding inside a pump.

This lowering of the central tendon is, however, rapidly **checked by the stretching of the mediastinal contents** but mainly by the presence of the **mass of the abdominal viscera.** From this moment (Fig. 27), the central tendon becomes the **fixed point** (large white arrow) and the muscle fibres, now acting from the margin of the central tendon, **elevate the lower ribs.** If the

point **P is taken as fixed** and the **rib as rotating about the centre O**, the extremity of the rib describes the **arc of a circle AB**, while the corresponding muscle fibres shorten by a length **A′B** (double white arrow). Thus, by elevating the lower ribs, the diaphragm *increases the transverse diameter of the lower thorax* and at the same time, with the help of the sternum, it also *elevates the upper ribs,* thereby increasing the thoracic anteroposterior diameter.

Therefore, it can be stated that the diaphragm is an **essential respiratory muscle**, since it *increases by itself the three diameters of the thoracic cavity:*

- **it increases the vertical diameter** by the lowering of the central tendon, which can be curtailed by an **increase in volume of the abdominal contents** owing to a build-up of intestinal gas (also known as abdominal meteorism), particularly common with **intestinal obstruction**
- **it increases the transverse diameter** by elevating the lower limbs
- **it increases the anteroposterior diameter** by elevating the upper ribs with the help of the sternum.

Its **significance in the physiology of respiration** is evident.

Hiccups are due to *spasmodic, rhythmical and repeated contractions of the diaphragm.* Their aetiology is poorly known, with two possible causes:

- a *central* cause related to irritation of the phrenic nerve
- a *peripheral* cause related to irritation of the dome of the diaphragm.

Hiccups are usually a transient problem and subside after a variable length of time. When they persist they are difficult to treat.

Fig. 25

Fig. 26

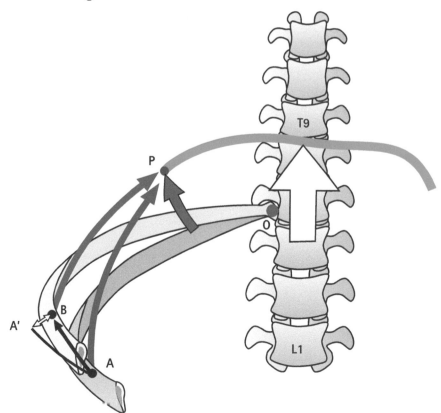

Fig. 27

The respiratory muscles

As we have already seen, the respiratory muscles fall into **two categories:**
- the **inspiratory muscles**, which elevate the ribs and the sternum
- the **expiratory muscles**, which depress the ribs and the sternum.

These two categories comprise **two groups** each, i.e. the **primary group** and the **accessory group** of muscles. The latter group is recruited only during **abnormally deep or strong respiratory movements.**

Therefore, the respiratory muscles can be subdivided into **four groups.**

First group

This includes the main inspiratory muscles, i.e. the **external intercostals**, the **levatores costarum** and **above all the diaphragm**.

Second group

This comprises the following **accessory inspiratory muscles** (Figs 28-30):
- the sternocleidomastoids (1) and the anterior (2), middle (3) and posterior (4) scalenes; these muscles are active in inspiration only when *they act from the cervical spine*, which must be kept rigid by other muscles (Fig. 28)
- the pectoralis major (16) and the pectoralis minor (5), when they act from the *shoulder girdle and the abducted upper limbs* (Fig. 30, inspired by Rodin's *Bronze Age*)
- the lower fibres of the serratus anterior (5) and the latissimus dorsi (10), when the latter acts from (Fig. 29) the *already abducted upper limb*

- the serratus posterior superior (11)
- the iliocostalis cervicis (12), inserted cranially into the last five cervical *transverse processes* and arising caudally from the *angles of the upper six ribs*. The direction of its fibres is almost the same as that of the *levatores costarum longi*.

Third group

This includes the **primary expiratory muscles**, i.e. the **internal intercostals**. In fact, normal expiration is a purely passive process due to the recoil of the thorax on itself as a result of the elasticity of its osteochondral components and of the pulmonary parenchyma. Thus the energy necessary for expiration is, in reality, derived from the **payback of the energy** generated by the inspiratory muscles and stored in the elastic components of the thorax and lungs. We shall see later the vital role played by the **costal cartilages** (see p. 179). Note also that in the erect position the ribs are pulled down by their own weight, and the contribution of gravity is not negligible.

Fourth group

This includes the **accessory expiratory muscles.** Though accessory, they are not less important and are extremely powerful. They underlie **forced expiration** and the **Valsalva manoeuvre.** The **abdominal muscles** (Fig. 30), i.e. the rectus abdominis (7), the external oblique (8) and the internal oblique (9) *strongly depress the thoracic outlet.*

The thoracolumbar region (Fig. 29) contains the other **accessory expiratory muscles**, i.e. the iliocostalis thoracis (13), the longissimus (14), the serratus posterior inferior (15) and the quadratus lumborum (not shown here).

Fig. 28

Fig. 29

Fig. 30

163

Antagonism-synergism between the diaphragm and the abdominal muscles

The diaphragm is the main inspiratory muscle. The abdominal muscles are extremely strong accessory expiratory muscles, which are essential to produce forced expiration and the Valsalva manoeuvre. Yet these muscles, which appear to be antagonistic, are synergistic at the same time. This may seem paradoxical and even illogical, but in practice they cannot function independently. This is an example of **antagonism-synergism.** What then is the functional relationship between the diaphragm and the abdominal muscles during the two phases of breathing?

During inspiration
During inspiration (Fig. 31, side view and Fig. 32, anterior view) contraction of the diaphragm *lowers the central tendon* (red arrows), thus *increasing the vertical diameter of the thorax*. These changes are soon opposed by the *stretching of the mediastinal contents* (M) and above all by the *resistance of the abdominal viscera* (R), which are held in place by the **abdominal girdle** formed by the **powerful abdominal muscles**, i.e. the rectus muscle (RA), the transversus muscle (T), and the internal (IO) and external (EO) obliques anteriorly. Without them the abdominal contents would be displaced inferiorly and anteriorly, and the *central tendon would not be able to provide a solid anchor for the diaphragm* **to elevate the ribs.** Thus this **antagonistic-synergistic action** of the abdominal muscles is essential for the efficiency of the diaphragm. This notion is borne out in disease, e.g. in *poliomyelitis, where paralysis of the abdominal muscles* reduces the ventilatory efficiency of the diaphragm. In Figure 31 (side view) the directions of the fibres of the large flat muscles of the abdomen represent a six-sided star, which is an oversimplified version of the 'woven texture' of the abdominal wall.

During expiration
During expiration (Fig. 33, side view and Fig. 34, anterior view) the diaphragm relaxes, and the contraction of the abdominal muscles lowers the lower ribs around the thoracic outlet, thereby *decreasing concurrently the transverse and antero-posterior diameters of the thorax*. Furthermore, by increasing the intra-abdominal pressure, they *push the viscera upwards* and raise the *central tendon*. **This decreases the vertical diameter of the thorax** and closes the costodiaphragmatic recesses. The abdominal muscles therefore are the **perfect antagonists of the diaphragm** because they *reduce simultaneously the three thoracic diameters*.

The respective roles of the diaphragm and of the abdominal muscles can be visualized **graphically** (Fig. 35) as follows. Both sets of muscles are in a state of permanent contraction, but their **tonic activity varies reciprocally.**

During inspiration the *tonus of the diaphragm increases, while that of the abdominal muscles decreases*. Conversely, **during expiration** the *tonus of the abdominal muscles increases while that of the diaphragm decreases*.

Hence there exists between these two muscle groups a **dynamic balance**, which *is constantly shifting one way or the other* and *provides an example of the concept of antagonism-synergism*.

The strong contraction of the main and accessory expiratory muscles on a **closed glottis** produces the so-called '**abdominal effort**', which transforms the abdomen into a '**pneumatic beam**', so important in the lifting of weights (see p. 20).

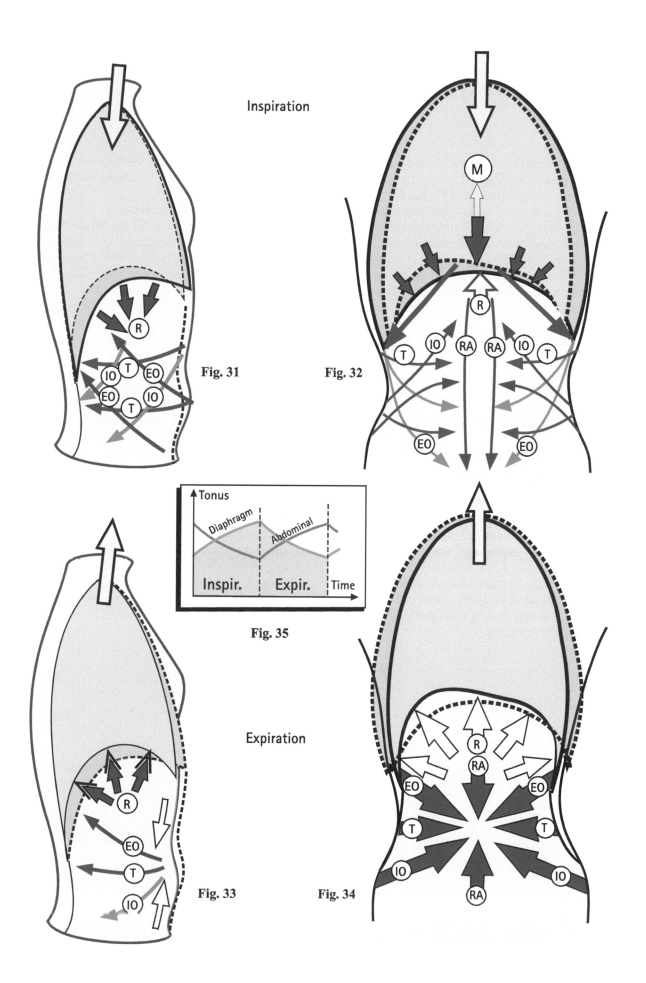

Inspiration

Fig. 31

Fig. 32

Tonus

Diaphragm

Abdominal

Inspir. Expir. Time

Fig. 35

Expiration

Fig. 33

Fig. 34

Airflow in the respiratory passages

Funck's classic experiment (Figs 36 and 37) demonstrates the flow of air in the respiratory passages. Replace the bottom of a flask by a watertight elastic membrane and put inside the flask a rubber balloon, which is connected to the outside by a tube going through a cork. The balloon can be inflated or deflated simply *by moving the elastic membrane. If this membrane is pulled down* (Fig. 37), the internal volume of the flask is increased by a volume **V**, while the internal pressure *falls below the atmospheric pressure*. As a result, a volume of air **exactly equal to V** enters the tube and *inflates the rubber balloon*. **This is the mechanism of inspiration.**

Conversely, if *the elastic membrane is released* (Fig. 36), it recoils and the volume of the flask decreases by *the same volume* V, while the internal pressure rises and the air inside the balloon is driven out through the tube. **This is the mechanism of expiration.**

Thus respiration depends on the **increase or decrease** in the volume of the thoracic cavity (Fig. 38). If initially the thorax is taken to be a **truncated ovoid** with base ACBD, transverse diameter CD, anteroposterior diameter AB and vertical diameter SP, then the action of the respiratory muscles, especially the diaphragm, increases all its diameters into those of a *greater truncated ovoid* A′C′B′D′, with an anteroposterior diameter A′B′, a transverse diameter C′D′ and a vertical diameter SP′. The only difference here from Funck's experiment lies in the fact that *all the dimensions of the container have increased simultaneously*. There are, however, **striking similarities between the experimental setup and the anatomical reality**, namely the following:

- the *vertical tube* for the passage of air is the trachea
- the *inflated balloon* is the lungs

- the *elastic membrane* at the bottom of the flask is the *diaphragm*, which also increases all the other diameters concerned.

Two points need to be emphasized:

- On the one hand the lungs **fill the whole thoracic cavity** and are connected to the thoracic wall by the potential **pleural space**, i.e. **the pleura**. In fact its two normally **apposed** layers glide freely one on the other and ensure a tight mechanical link between the lungs and the thoracic cavity without limiting the respiratory movements, as the lungs dilate and *move relative to the thoracic wall*.
- On the other hand, during inspiration, the intrathoracic pressure falls and becomes negative, not only with respect to the outside but also *with respect to the abdominal cavity*. As a result, air enters the trachea and the pulmonary alveoli, and **venous return to the right atrium** (RA) **is speeded up**. Thus inspiration **improves cardiac filling** and, with the help of the lesser circulation, **it brings venous blood into close contact** with fresh, newly inspired air in the alveoli. **Thus inspiration at once ensures air entry and pulmonary vascular perfusion.**

In terms of respiratory airflow let us consider **snoring**, which is often very unpleasant for one's bedmate. *Almost all human beings snore – and even some animals –* but there are certain *structural types* and *positions* that predispose to this infirmity. Snoring is produced by *vibrations of the soft palate* taking place in the supine position and during deep sleep. There are now some more or less efficacious medical treatments; occasionally, only surgical palatoplasty can be curative.

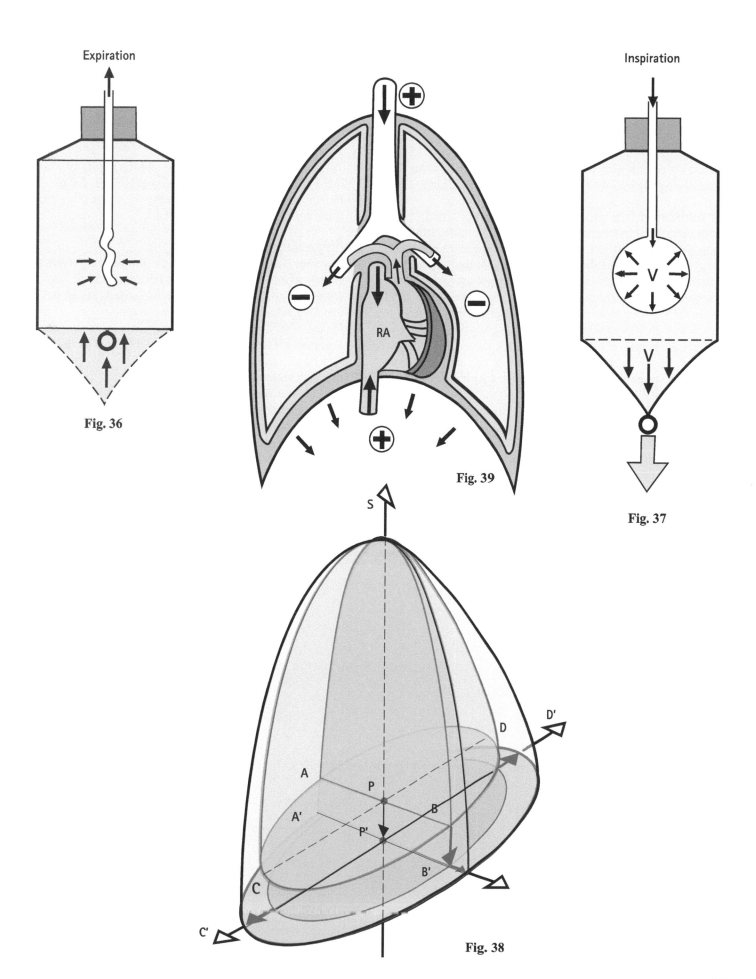

Expiration

Fig. 36

Inspiration

Fig. 37

Fig. 39

RA

Fig. 38

S

Respiratory volumes

Respiratory or pulmonary volumes are the volumes of air displaced during the various phases and types of breathing.

Comparison of the various respiratory volumes

We find it helpful to represent these various volumes using the pleats of an accordion, as it simplifies comparison among them.

- **During quiet breathing at rest** (Fig. 40) the various respiratory volumes can be defined as follows: the air displaced between normal inspiration and normal expiration is the **tidal volume** (TV, i.e. 500 mL). In the diagram this volume is shown as the blue-tinted band (2) containing the *oscillations of the spirogram*.
- If normal inspiration is prolonged by a forced inspiration, the extra volume inhaled represents the **inspiratory reserve volume** (IRV, i.e. 1.5 L).
- The sum of the inspiratory reserve volume and of the tidal volume is the **inspiratory capacity** (IC, i.e. 2 L).
- If a normal expiration is prolonged to the maximum by a forced expiration, the volume exhaled is the **expiratory reserve volume** (ERV, i.e. 1.5 L).
- The sum of the inspiratory reserve volume, the tidal volume and the expiratory reserve volume is the **vital capacity** (VC, i.e. 3.5 L).
- Even after a complete expiration some air cannot be expelled and is still present in the lungs and in the bronchi, i.e. the **residual volume** (RV, i.e. 0.5 L).

- The sum of the residual volume and the expiratory volume is the **functional reserve capacity** (FRC, i.e. 2 L).
- Finally, the sum of the vital capacity and the residual volume is the **total lung capacity** (i.e. 4 L).

During exercise

During exercise (Fig. 41) the various volumes are *broken down differently* within the total lung capacity, as follows:

- *Only the residual volume is unchanged*, as it can never be expelled, whatever the force of expiration.
- On the other hand, as the respiratory rate increases, **the tidal volume** (TV) **rises to a maximum**, but then as the respiratory rate increases the *tidal volume tends to fall slightly*. Thus the *tidal volume does attain a maximum*.
- The expiratory reserve volume increases markedly, indicating that the *depth of rapid breathing during exercise* comes closer to the level of maximal distension of the thorax than during breathing at rest.
- As a result of the increase in tidal volume and of the expiratory reserve volume, **the inspiratory reserve volume drops** (IRV). In Figure 41 the spirogram at rest has been added for comparison.

All these details are quite logical, easy to remember and of great importance in daily efforts and sports activities.

Fig. 40

Fig. 41

The physiopathology of breathing

Many factors can interfere with respiratory efficiency.

The problem of the **flail chest** can be illustrated by a **modified Funck's experiment** (Fig. 42). If part of the wall of the flask is replaced by another elastic membrane, it follows that, when the bottom membrane is pulled down, the membrane in the wall of the flask is **sucked in and displaces a volume v, which must be subtracted from the total volume V.** Therefore, the inflated balloon has a smaller volume **V minus v.**

In humans the **flail chest** is the result of a violent blow to the thorax; as a result, a fairly large part of the thoracic wall **stops following its movements and is sucked in during inspiration**, leading to **paradoxical respiration.** Respiratory efficiency is reduced, leading to **respiratory distress** with a catastrophic drop in *the oxygen uptake in the alveolar capillaries.*

There are also many other conditions associated with reduced respiratory efficiency and even culminating in *respiratory distress.* They are mostly due to ventilatory problems and are summarized in Figure 43.

- **Pneumothorax** (1) is the entry of air into the pleural cavity, followed by recoil of the lung by its own elasticity (2). It can be caused by a pleuropulmonary tear, where at every inspiration (black arrow) air enters the pleural cavity. This corresponds to **traumatopnoea**, which leads to severe respiratory distress. The entry of air into the pleural space can also result from the rupture of a **bronchus** or of an **emphysematous bulla.** When the pleura no longer pulls on the lung, the latter becomes useless (2). This can also result from a **haemothorax** (blood in the pleural cavity), a **hydrothorax** (fluid in the pleural cavity) or **pleurisy** (3), when the fluid gathers at the base of the thorax.
- **Flail chest** (4) also causes a more or less severe loss of respiratory efficiency.
- In **bronchial obstruction with atelectasis** (5) the territory supplied by the bronchus receives no air and the lung tissue

retracts. In the diagram the left upper lobe is **atelectatic** owing to obstruction of the upper lobe bronchus.

- In **inflammatory pleural thickening** (6) following a pleurisy, a pyothorax or a haemothorax, the **shell-like sclerotic pleura** hugs the lung tightly and *prevents it from expanding during inspiration.*
- **Acute gastric dilatation** (7) hinders the descent of the diaphragm.
- **Severe intestinal distension due to obstruction** (8) displaces the diaphragm upwards; it is an **abdominal cause** of respiratory distress.
- **Phrenic nerve palsy** (Fig. 44) can interfere with breathing. In the diagram, interruption of the left phrenic nerve leads to **paralysis of the left hemidiaphragm**, which exhibits paradoxical respiratory movements, e.g. up instead of down during inspiration.

Ventilatory mechanics can also be altered considerably by **the position of the body.**

- **In the supine position** (Fig. 45) the weight of the abdominal viscera pushes the diaphragm upwards, making *inspiration more difficult.* The tidal volume is reduced and displaced upwards in the diagram (Fig. 43), at the expense of the inspiratory reserve volume. This occurs **under general anaesthesia** and can be made worse by anaesthetic drugs and muscle relaxants, which reduce the efficiency of the respiratory muscles. Hence the value of assisted breathing after tracheal intubation, normally administered by the anaesthetist or mechanically using a respirator. It also occurs in the **comatose patient.**
- **When the subject lies on one side** (Fig. 46), the diaphragm is pushed upwards far more on the lower side. The **lower lung is less efficient** than the upper lung and, to make matters worse, circulatory stasis supervenes. Anaesthetists particularly dread this position.

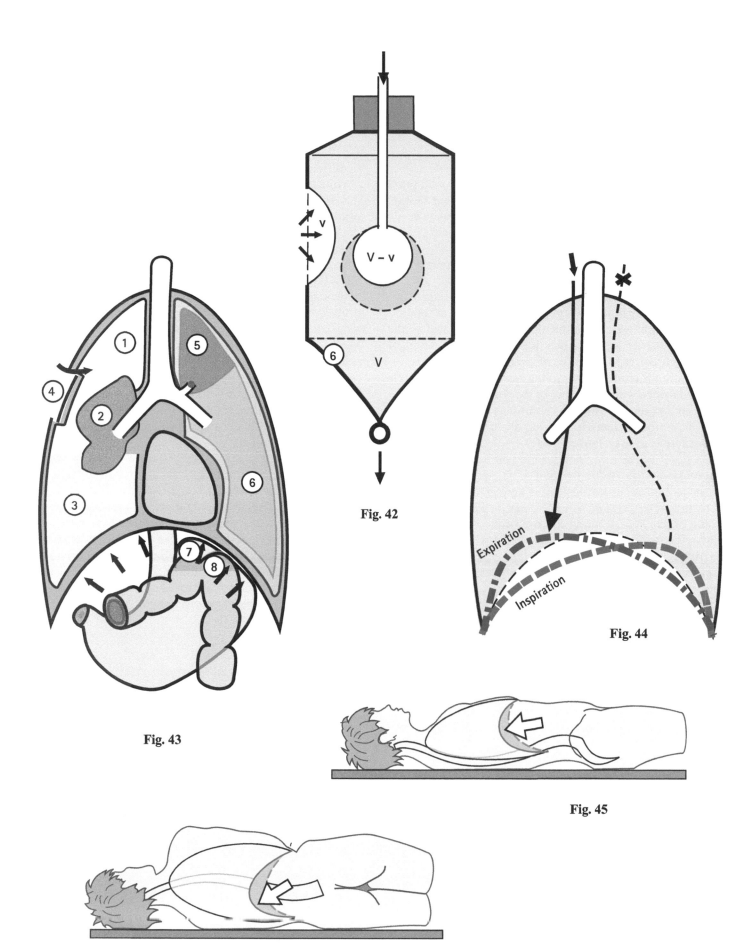

Fig. 42

Fig. 43

Fig. 44

Fig. 45

Fig. 46

Respiratory types: athletes, musicians and others...

Ventilatory mechanics varies with **age and sex** (Fig. 47):
- **in women**, breathing is mostly upper thoracic, with maximum range of movement occurring in the upper thorax, which shows an increase in its anteroposterior diameter
- **in men**, it is **mixed**, i.e. **upper and lower thoracic**
- **in the child**, it is **abdominal**
- **in the aged** it is greatly altered by the development of a thoracic kyphosis.

To understand the respiratory pathophysiology of the aged, reference to a **Chinese lantern** (Fig. 48) can be helpful as follows:
- In this *thought experiment* the thorax is represented by the Chinese lantern hanging on one side from a rigid and straight rod, which corresponds to the *thoracic spine*.
- **Inspiration** is produced by **pulling on the uppermost circle of the lantern**, corresponding to the contraction of the scalene and sternocleidomastoid muscles. At the same time the bottom of the lantern is pulled down, corresponding to **contraction of the diaphragm** (D).
- As a result of these two actions the **volume of the lantern increases** and air rushes inside it.
- If the pull on the uppermost circle and on the bottom of the lantern is released (Fig. 49), the lantern collapses under the force of gravity (g) along the rigid rod corresponding to the spine, and its volume decreases. This is equivalent to **expiration.**
- Let us now assume that the supporting rod is **not straight but curved** (Fig. 50), as *in a kyphotic spine*. The lantern stays forever in a collapsed and deflated state, and it is much more difficult to pull the uppermost circle upwards. Therefore the volume **R** does not contribute to ventilation.

This experiment illustrates the **respiratory difficulties caused by an accentuated thoracic curvature, i.e. thoracic kyphosis**. The same problems arise **in the aged** (Fig. 51). The increased upper thoracic curvature brings the ribs closer together and reduces the range of their movements. Thus the upper lobes of the lungs are poorly aerated, and breathing becomes lower thoracic or even abdominal. This state of affairs is made worse by the hypotonicity of the muscles. The loss of elasticity in the costal cartilages also contributes to a drop in the tidal volume. When dealing with the physiology of breathing, the **sigh** deserves mention; it is the result of a *deep inspiration* followed by a *prolonged expiration*. Physiologically it helps to renew the air in the dead space and in the reserve compartments. Psychologically this quasi-unconscious act *relieves emotional tension*, particularly anxiety, which is generally speaking dissipated by the *sigh of relief after an ordeal*.

Breathing plays a major role in some professions e.g. **athletics**, and in particular **swimming**. It is also vital for **musicians playing wind instruments** and **singers**, who need maximal **respiratory capacity and control of the breath, so dependent on the control of the expiratory muscles**. Moreover, among musicians at large, breathing plays an important role outside its ventilatory function, since *its rhythm shapes the very performance of the musician*. In certain adagios the breathing pattern is so distinct that *it can be said to act as an internal metronome for the musician*.

M. Sternocleidomastoid

Air

M. Scalenes

M

Inspiration

D

Fig. 48

Fig. 47

Air

Expiration

g

Fig. 49

R

Kyphosis

Fig. 50

Fig. 51

173

The dead space

The dead space is the volume of air that *does not contribute to respiratory* exchange. In Figure 52 the respiratory volumes are represented by the accordion. If the exhaust pipe is extended by a **sizable container** (DS) the *dead space is artificially increased.* In fact, if only the tidal volume of 500 ml is being displaced, and if the combined volume of tube and container is also 500 ml, then breathing will only displace air within the dead space and *no fresh air will move inside the accordion.*

The case of the diver (Fig. 53) is even easier to grasp. Let us assume that he is connected to the surface only by a tube through which he inhales and exhales. If the tube volume equals his vital capacity he will never be able to inhale fresh air, despite his most energetic efforts. *Whenever he takes a breath, he will only inhale the air polluted by his own previous expiration.* Thus **he will soon die of asphyxia**, as occasionally happened in the early days of diving. This problem is solved by conveying fresh air through a tube and by allowing the expired air to be expelled by **a valve placed in the helmet**, as evidenced by the bubbles.

The anatomical dead space (Fig. 54) is **the volume of the respiratory tree**, i.e. the **upper airways**, including mouth and nose, the trachea, the bronchi and the bronchioles. This volume equals 150 ml, so that during normal breathing, *when only the tidal volume is displaced*, no more than **350 ml of fresh air** participates in alveolar gas exchange and *oxygenation of venous blood*. Efficiency is improved by:

- increasing the volume of air displaced by recruiting the inspiratory or expiratory reserve volume, or
- decreasing the volume of the dead space as with a **tracheotomy** (T), which connects the trachea directly to the outside and cuts down the dead space by nearly a half.

Tracheotomy, however, is not without risks, as it *deprives the respiratory tree of its natural defences*, i.e. filtration and warming of inspired air by the nasal fossae and above all closure of the glottis against foreign bodies, and exposes it to **severe bronchopulmonary infections.** It must therefore be used only in cases of severe and immediate danger.

In Figure 55 the **respiratory volumes are represented by the accordion** and the tracheotomy by the opening at the base of the tube (see also Figs 40 and 41, page 169).

There is **another type of dead space** (Fig. 56), i.e. the **physiological dead space** (PDS), which results **from the loss of vascular perfusion of a pulmonary segment from a pulmonary embolus** (PE). **Ventilation of this unperfused segment is wasted**, thereby increasing the anatomical dead space.

PE

PDS

Fig. 56

IRV
VC
ERV

RV

Fig. 55

DS

Fig. 52

Fig. 53

T

Fig. 54

175

Thoracic compliance

Compliance is related directly to the *elasticity of the anatomical component* of the thorax and the lungs.

In normal expiration (Fig. 57) the thorax and the lungs regain their position of equilibrium, which can be compared to that of a spring at rest. Thus the intra-alveolar pressure and the atmospheric pressure are in equilibrium.

During forced expiration (Fig. 58) the active muscles *compress the elastic components* of the thorax. To use a concrete example, if the *spring* representing the thorax is compressed to generate a **positive intrathoracic pressure** of +20 cm of water, the intrapulmonary pressure will exceed the atmospheric pressure and air will escape through the trachea. Meanwhile the thorax *will tend to regain its original position* even as the spring will tend to go back to its **original position 0.**

Conversely, **during forced inspiration** (Fig. 59), which could be compared to *stretching of the spring*, a **negative pressure** of −20 cm of water develops in the thorax relative to the atmospheric pressure. As a result, air enters the trachea, but *the elasticity of the thorax will again tend to bring it back to its original position*. These changes can be **represented graphically** by using **compliance curves** (Fig. 60), which *relate the change in intrathoracic pressure (abscissa) to the changes in intrathoracic volume (ordinate).*

Three such curves can be drawn:

- **The curve for total thoracic relaxation** (T), where zero pressure corresponds to the volume at total relaxation (VR), and is the resultant of the volume/pressure curve for the lungs alone (L) and of the volume/pressure curve of the thoracic wall alone (W).

It is remarkable that the residual volume corresponds to the point where the pressure exerted by the elasticity of the thoracic wall (PW) and that exerted by the elasticity of the lungs (PL) are equal and opposite.

- **At volume V3**, i.e. at 70% of total lung capacity, the pressure generated purely by the thoracic wall is zero, and the pressure generated at total relaxation of the thorax is entirely due to the elasticity of the lungs (the two curves **L** and **T** intersect at this point).

- **At an intermediate volume** (VR) the pressure generated purely by relaxation of the thoracic wall is exactly equal to one half of the pressure generated by relaxation of the lungs. Thus the pressure generated by total relaxation of the thoracic wall is equal to one half of the pressure generated by relaxation of the lungs.

A final point deserves emphasis. *At maximal expiration the lungs have not yet lost all their elasticity* because the curve **L** is still to the right of zero pressure. This explains why when air is allowed to enter the pleural spaces the lungs can still retract to a minimum volume **Vp**, at which point they cannot retract any more and therefore exert no pressure on the air they still contain.

The total elasticity of the thorax (Fig. 61) can be compared to a **combination of two springs** (A): a large spring **W** representing the thoracic wall and a small spring **L** representing the lungs. The functional dependence of the lungs on the thoracic wall via the pleura can be represented by the coupling of the two springs (B), which requires *compressing the large spring* **W** and *stretching the small spring* **L**. The coupling of these two springs is equivalent to a single spring (C), which represents the total elasticity of the thorax (T); however, if the functional link between lung and thoracic wall is destroyed, each spring regains its own position of equilibrium (A).

To summarize, compliance is the *relationship between the volume of air and the wall pressure needed to displace it*. In the graph (Fig. 60) compliance corresponds to the slope of the middle of each curve so that the slope of the green curve (the compliance of the lungs) is greater than that of the blue curve (the compliance of the thoracic wall), and the total thoracic compliance is the algebraic sum of these two compliances (red curve).

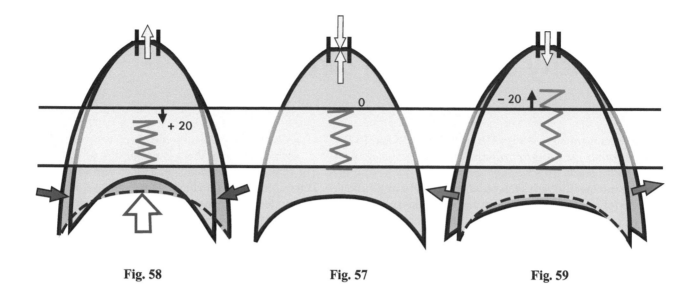

Fig. 58 Fig. 57 Fig. 59

Fig. 60

Fig. 61

177

The elasticity of the costal cartilages

As already demonstrated (see Figs 19 and 20, pp. 155 and 157), *during inspiration the costal cartilages undergo angular displacement and torsion around their long axes*. This torsion is important in the **mechanism of expiration.** During inspiration (I) the posterior ends of the ribs stay attached to the spine at the joints of costal heads (Fig. 62) and, as the sternum rises, the costal cartilages **rotate on their long axes** as indicated by the arrows t and t′.

At the same time, **the angles at the costochondral and sternocostal joints are altered.** (To make this easier to understand, the diagram shows the sternum as fixed and the spine as movable, which is mechanically a similar arrangement.)

Diagrammatically, the costochondral and sternocostal joints (Fig. 63) are **interlocking joints** at each end of the cartilage:

- **The medial end of the cartilage** (3) and the **sternal border** (1) are tightly interlocked, forming a **solid angle** (2), completely filled by the tip of the cartilage (4). This allows some movement vertically but **no torsion at all.**
- **The lateral end of the cartilage** (5) is shaped like a **cone flattened anteroposteriorly** and *fits snugly into the anterior end of the rib* (6), *which is correspondingly shaped to receive it.* Here again some lateral and vertical displacements are possible, but there is **no torsion at all.**

The opposite movements take place during expiration (E).

During inspiration (Fig. 64), when the rib is lowered relative to the sternum, which rises, the costal cartilage *twists on its own axis through an angle* **t**, and thus behaves like a **torsion rod**, which resembles a *spring that works not by shortening and lengthening but by torsion, as the name indicates.* This device, well known to engineers, is used as a shock-absorber in cars. Thus, if a rod is twisted on its long axis, its elasticity stores the torsion energy and releases it when the twisting stops. Likewise, the energy generated by the inspiratory muscles is **stored in the torsion bars of the costal cartilages** during inspiration; when these muscles start to relax, the elasticity of these cartilages suffices to bring the **thoracic skeleton back to its initial position.** The flexibility and elasticity of these cartilages decrease with age and eventually they tend to ossify, leading to a **loss of thoracic flexibility and respiratory efficiency in the aged.**

This mechanical analysis brings out the *important role played by the elastic costal cartilages in connecting the rigid ribs to the mobile sternum.*

Fig. 62

Fig. 63

Fig. 64

179

The mechanism of coughing and the Heimlich manoeuvre

Mechanism of coughing

As air enters the respiratory passages, it is **filtered, humidified and warmed up** by the nasal fossae and becomes theoretically free of **suspended particles** when it enters the trachea and the bronchi. However, if by accident, **foreign particles** gain access to the bronchial tree, there is a very efficient mechanism designed to remove them – **coughing.** Similarly, coughing is designed to expel **packets of bronchial mucous secretions**, which trap these fine particles and are then wafted towards the glottis by the **constant ciliary activity of the bronchial epithelium** – *an activity severely compromised by smoking.*

The mechanism of coughing has three phases:

- **Phase 1** (Fig. 65) is the **inspiratory phase** or the so-called preparatory phase, when the bulk of the **respiratory reserve volume** is drawn into the bronchial tree and alveoli. The disadvantage of this deep inspiration it that it can carry down towards the bronchioles any foreign bodies lying below the glottis.
- **Phase II** (Fig. 66) is the **pressure phase**, which involves **closure of the glottis** and violent contraction of the **intercostal muscles** and of all the *accessory expiratory muscles*, particularly the **abdominal muscles.** During this phase there is a **sharp rise in intrathoracic pressure.**
- **Phase III** (Fig. 67) is the **expulsion phase.** While the accessory expiratory muscles are still contracted, **the glottis opens suddenly** and violently releases **a current of air** from the bronchial tree. This carries along the foreign particles and the packets of mucus **past the open glottis** towards the **pharynx**, whence they **are coughed up from the oropharynx.**

Therefore, it appears that the **efficiency** of coughing depends on:

- recruitment of the efficient **abdominal muscles** (thus coughing is *inefficient or impossible* in **patients with poliomyelitis** and abdominal wall paralysis and even **after abdominal operations**, when any contraction of these muscles is painful and feared)
- **closure of the glottis** requiring the **integrity of the laryngeal muscles and of its neural control.**

Coughing is a **reflex act** set off by sensory receptors located at the **tracheal bifurcation** (the carina) and in the **pleura.** The afferent fibres of this reflex are carried centrally in the **vagus nerves** to the **bulbar** centres; its efferent fibres are carried not only by the **laryngeal nerves**, which are branches of the vagus nerves, but also by the **intercostal and abdominal nerves.** Its delicately balanced mechanism can easily be upset.

The Heimlich manoeuvre

There are situations **when coughing is inappropriate**, for example when **a large foreign body** has been inhaled. This happens when an adult, trying to swallow a badly chewed piece of meat, forces it down the wrong way. The mouthful unexpectedly gets past the protective mechanisms of the respiratory tract and ends up in the trachea. Children can inhale sweets or a piece of brioche in the same way. **It is a dramatic event**, since the subject tries to take a deep breath in order to cough and only manages to **drive the foreign object farther down his trachea**, which makes his respiratory distress worse. Without immediate help from outside he can die of **acute asphyxia.** People should know the **life-saving procedures** in such unfortunate situations:

- Hold a child who is not too big upside down by its feet and shake it so as to dislodge the sweet.
- Deliver a series of strong thumps to the back of an adult; however, if there is no improvement after five thumps, proceed to more effective life-saving procedures.
- The **Heimlich manoeuvre** (Fig. 68), well known to first-aid workers, consists of violently compressing the epigastrium of the subject in distress while standing behind him.
- The manoeuvre can be performed on oneself, if alone, by compressing the epigastrium on the back of a chair.
- This manoeuvre should be taught to all babysitters, young parents and students in medicine and physical therapy in their first year of study.

Fig. 65

Fig. 66

Fig. 67

Fig. 68

The laryngeal muscles and the protection of the airways during swallowing

The highly sophisticated **laryngeal apparatus**, the gateway to the trachea, has three essential functions:

- **closure of the glottis** during the **Valsalva manoeuvre** and **coughing**
- **protection of the airways** during swallowing
- **phonation.**

Understanding these functions requires a review of the anatomy of the larynx. A **posterior oblique view** (Fig. 69) shows the following **cartilages** joined to one another:

- The signet-ring-shaped **cricoid cartilage** (6), corresponding to the first ring of the trachea, has a **signet plate*** (see Fig. 75, p. 185) or posterior lamina (7) with **two articular facets**, one on each side: the **thyroid or inferior facet** (22), articulating with the inferior horn of the thyroid cartilage (5), and the **arytenoid or superior facet** (21), articulating with the arytenoid cartilage (8).

- The **thyroid cartilage**: its **medial surface** (2) is visible, but its lateral surface is obscured by the **oblique line** (3), which bears on the **superior part of its posterior border** the **superior horns** (4), attached to the **hyoid bone** (not shown here) by the **thyrohyoid ligaments**. It consists of **two laminae** forming a solid angle open anteriorly. The inferior part of its posterior surface (see Fig. 76, p. 185) receives the **anterior attachments** (26) of the vocal cords (15).

The **roughly pyramidal arytenoid cartilages** (8), lying on either side of the signet plate of the cricoid cartilage, have three processes:

- a **superior process** or corniculate cartilage (23) (see Figs 75 and 76, p. 185)
- a medial or **vocal process** (25) giving attachment to the vocal cord
- a lateral or **muscular process** giving insertion to the posterior crico-arytenoid muscle (13 and 14).

Between the corniculate cartilage and the upper border of the signet plate of the cricoid cartilage runs a **Y-shaped ligament**, i.e. the **cricocorniculate ligament** (12), which carries a **small cartilaginous nodule**, i.e. the **interarytenoid cartilage** (11) at the junction of its **lower stem** and its **two upper branches** (10). The **stalk of the epiglottic cartilage** (1) is attached to the posterior aspect of the solid angle formed by the thyroid laminae. Shaped like a leaf, it is concave posteriorly and its long axis is oblique superoinferiorly. Its two lateral edges are attached to the corniculate cartilage by the **two aryepiglottic ligaments** (9).

Also seen (Fig. 69, p. 183 and Fig. 73, p. 185) are the **right lateral cricoarytenoid muscle** (16), which unites the *muscular process of the arytenoid* and the *anterior part of the arch of the cricoid*, and the **right cricothyroid muscle** (17) running between the *inferior border of the thyroid cartilage and the anterior border of the cricoid arch*.

In Figure 70 the **laryngeal inlet** is marked by an arrow and is bounded as follows:

- superiorly by the **epiglottic cartilage** (1)
- laterally by the **aryepiglottic ligaments** (9), reinforced by the **aryepiglottic muscles** (19)
- inferiorly by the **corniculate cartilages** (23), united by the **cricorniculate ligaments** (10), which are reinforced posteriorly by the transverse fibres of the **transverse interarytenoid muscles** (18).

The lateral walls of this inlet are completed by the superficial fibres of the **inferior thyroarytenoid muscles** (20). The inlet is shown open as in normal breathing.

During swallowing the glottis is closed, and the epiglottis tilts inferiorly and posteriorly (Fig. 71) towards the corniculate cartilages by the pull of the **aryepiglottic muscles** (19) and **the inferior thyroarytenoid muscles** (20). Solid and liquid foods slide down on the **anterosuperior surface of the epiglottis** towards the oropharynx and the **entrance to the oesophagus** (not shown) lying posterior to the cricoid.

---

* This term comes from its resemblance to the wider uppermost part of a signet ring.

Fig. 69

Fig. 70

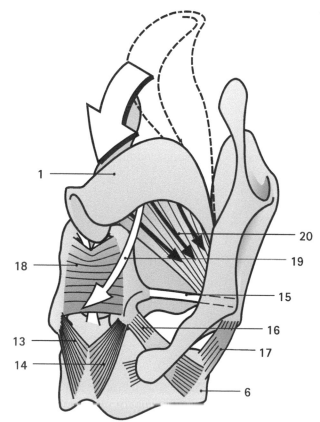

Fig. 71

The glottis and the vocal cords: phonation

The glottis is the passage that controls the flow of air in the larynx. **Two diagrams** (Figs 72 and 73, superior view) explain how the glottis functions.

The rima glottidis seen from the pharynx, i.e. from above, is a **triangular fissure with an anterior apex** (Fig. 72), and its two borders consist of the following:

- the **vocal cords** (15) joining the **posterior surface of the thyroid cartilage** (3) and the **vocal process** (25) of the arytenoid
- the **arytenoid cartilages** (24), which articulate from above with the **cricoid cartilage** (7) by two joints with two vertical axes o and o′.

Contraction of the **posterior cricoarytenoid muscles** (13) rotates the arytenoid cartilages on their axes o and o′ and abducts the vocal processes (25) *with opening of the glottis.*

Conversely (Fig. 73), when the **lateral cricoarytenoid muscles contract** (16), the arytenoid cartilages rotate in the opposite direction. The **vocal processes** (25) approach each other towards the midline, and the **vocal cords** (15′) come to touch each other, ensuring **closure of the rima glottidis.**

The **partial diagram of the vocal cords** (Fig. 74) shows that, when the glottis moves from the open (g) to the closed (g′) position, the vocal cords move from the open (15) to the closed (15′) position and are stretched for a length **d** by the displacements (red arrow) of the vocal processes caused by rotation of the arytenoid cartilages (24). The **increased tension** in the cords **produces a higher note during speech.**

The last two diagrams illustrate **how the glottis is closed** (Fig. 75) and how the **vocal cords are tensed** (Fig. 76) during speech.

A left **anterior view** (Fig. 75) of the **cricoid** (6) and **arytenoid** (8) **cartilages** shows the arytenoid resting on top of the signet plate of the cricoid (7), with which it articulates at the **arytenoid facet** (21). The axis of this **cricoarytenoid joint of synovial type** runs obliquely inferosuperiorly, mediolaterally and posterolaterally (not shown).

When the **interarytenoid** (18) and the **posterior cricoarytenoid** (14) muscles contract (see Fig. 71, p. 183), the arytenoid *swings laterally* to a new position (deep blue, Fig. 75), and its **vocal process** (25) *moves away from the midline.* The two **vocal cords** (15) form a *triangular orifice with an anteriorly located apex* (Fig. 72). Conversely, when the **lateral cricoarytenoid muscles contract** (Fig. 70, 16), the arytenoid cartilage swings *medially,* and its *vocal process approaches the midline as does the vocal cord* (15′) (Fig. 73).

During speech the vocal cords are subjected to varying tensions, as is well illustrated by the diagram (Fig. 74). On closure of the glottis the vocal cord is lengthened. Moreover (Fig. 76), assuming that the cricoid cartilage (6) stays put, **contraction of the cricothyroid** ((see Figs. 69-70-71) 17) rotates the thyroid cartilage around the axis of the joint between the inferior horn of the thyroid cartilage and the cricoid (5), so that its anterior part is lowered. The anterior insertion of the vocal cord **moves from position 26 to position 26′**, and the cord is lengthened as it is **actively stretched by the contracting cricothyroid** (17′). This muscle, innervated by the **recurrent laryngeal nerve**, is **therefore the most important muscle in speech**, since it *controls the tension in the vocal cords and hence the pitch of the sound.* There are thus two mechanisms that regulate the tension of the vocal cords:

- closure of the rima glottidis by contraction of the lateral cricoarytenoid muscle
- forward tilting of the thyroid cartilage by contraction of the cricothyroid muscle.

Fig. 72

Fig. 73

Fig. 74

Fig. 75

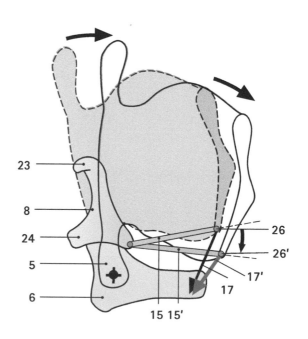

Fig. 76

Chapter 5

THE CERVICAL SPINE

The cervical spine is the uppermost segment of the spinal column continuous with the thoracic spine. It supports the head and forms the **skeleton of the neck.**

It is the **most mobile part** of the spine and has the task of **orienting the head** in an almost 180° sector of space both vertically and transversely. It must be stressed that **the mobility of the cervical spine and that of the eyeballs are additive.** Since the head contains the *main sensory organs* – **the eyes, the ears and the nose** – it must be able to localize potential threats to individuals and points of interest for their survival.

The **sagittal plane of the head** demarcates **two hemispaces,** i.e. right and left. Stimuli coming from these two hemispaces need to be separated to achieve **three-dimensional vision and hearing** and provide essential data for the localization of threats or points of interest. The neck is thus the equivalent of *radar supports* that rotate through space continuously. The only difference is that neck rotation cannot exceed 170-180°, which is already appreciable when compared to animals without necks, as for example fish, which, despite the great mobility of their eyes, must rotate their bodies in order to orient their sensors. As the most mobile segment of the spinal column, the cervical spine is also the **most fragile,** not only because of its mobility but also because of the lightness of its structural components, which only need to support the relatively low weight of the head, except when it has to support heavy loads, as is the case in some populations.

The neck, whose slenderness is of great aesthetic value in women, is the **most exposed part of the human body** and highly susceptible to deadly attacks by compression, strangulation, twisting or severing. The cervical spine must be handled with great care **after an accident,** and also during *all forms of treatment directed to it.*

The cervical spine taken as a whole

Taken as a whole (Fig. 1) the cervical spine is made up of **two anatomically and functionally distinct segments:**

- **the upper or suboccipital segment** (1) comprising the first cervical vertebra or the **atlas** and the second cervical vertebra or the **axis**; these vertebrae are connected to each other and to the **occipital bone** by an *articular complex* with **three axes and three degrees of freedom**
- **the lower segment** (2) stretching from the inferior surface of the **axis** to the superior surface of **the first thoracic vertebra** (T1).

The cervical vertebrae are all alike, except for the atlas and the axis, which differ from each other and from the other cervical vertebrae. The joints of the lower segment have only two types **of movement**, i.e. **flexion-extension** and **combined lateral flexion-rotation**, but *there are no pure movements of lateral flexion or rotation.*

Functionally these two segments are **complementary** in order to allow **pure movements of rotation, lateral flexion and flexion-extension** of the head. We shall see that there is an **antagonism-synergism relationship** between these two parts of the spinal column.

Fig. 1

Diagrammatic representation of the first three cervical vertebrae

These *highly simplified* diagrams illustrate the following vertebrae one on top of the other and in the same vertical plane:

- the atlas (Fig. 2)
- the axis (Fig. 3)
- the third cervical vertebra (Fig. 4).

The atlas

The **atlas** (Fig. 2) is **ring-shaped**, with its transverse diameter greater than its anteroposterior diameter. It has **two lateral masses** (1 and 1'), oval in shape with their long axes running obliquely anteriorly and medially, and each of these in turn bears:

- a **biconcave superior articular facet** (2 and 2'), facing superiorly and medially and articulating with the occipital condyles
- an **anteroposteriorly convex inferior articular facet**, facing inferiorly and medially and articulating with the superior facet of the axis (12 and 12').

Its **anterior arch** (3) has on its posterior aspect a **small oval-shaped cartilaginous articular facet** (4) articulating with the **dens axis** (11). **Its posterior arch** (5) is at first flattened superoinferiorly but becomes wider posteriorly to form not a *spinous process* but a **vertical crest, i.e. the posterior tubercle** (6) in the midline. Its **transverse processes** (7 and 7') are pierced by the **vertebral arteries** (8), which run in **deep grooves** (8') *behind the lateral masses.*

The axis

The **superior surface** (10) of the **body** (9) of the **axis** (Fig. 3) bears centrally the **dens** (11), which acts as a *pivot for the atlanto-axial joint,* and laterally **two articular facets** (12 and 12'), which overhang the body like *two shoulder pads,* face superiorly and laterally and are **convex anteroposteriorly and flat transversely.**

The **posterior arch** (16) is made up of two **narrow laminae** (13 and 15') running obliquely posteriorly and medially. The **spinous process** (18) has **two tubercles** like every other cervical vertebra. Below the **pedicle** (16) are attached the **inferior articular processes** (17 and 17'), with two **cartilage-coated**

articular facets, which are directed inferiorly and anteriorly and articulate with the **superior facets** of C3 (24 and 24'). The **transverse processes** (13 and 13') have each a **vertical foramen** (14) for the vertebral artery, i.e. the foramen transversarium.

The third cervical vertebra (C3)

C3 (Fig. 4) is similar to the last four cervical vertebrae and as such is a typical **cervical vertebra.** It has a **vertebral body** (9) shaped like a *parallelepiped,* which is wider than it is high. Its **superior discal surface** (20) is bordered on both sides by the **uncinate processes** (22 and 22'), which bear two facets *facing superiorly and medially* and articulate with two *flat facets located on either side of the inferior surface of the axis.*

The anterior border of its superior surface also has a **flat facet** (21), which faces superiorly and anteriorly and articulates with the posterior aspect of *a beak-like projection from the anterior border of the axis.*

Its **inferior discal surface** is bordered on both sides by **the articular facets of the uncovertebral joints**, facing *inferiorly and laterally*; it carries a *prominent beak-like* projection facing anteriorly and inferiorly.

The **posterior arch** of this typical cervical vertebra has two **articular processes** (23 and 23'), each with:

- a **superior facet** (24 and 24') facing superiorly and posteriorly and articulating with the **inferior facet of the overlying vertebra,** i.e. the inferior facet of the axis (17)
- an **inferior facet** (not visible in the diagram), directed inferiorly and anteriorly and articulating with the **superior facet** of C4.

Each **articular process** is connected to the vertebral body by the **pedicle** (25), which receives the **base of the transverse process** (26 and 26'), also attached to the **lateral surface of the body.** The latter has the shape of a **superiorly concave groove**, which is pierced near the vertebral body by a **round foramen** (29) for the **vertebral artery.** The transverse process terminates in **an anterior and a posterior tubercle.** The **vertebral laminae** (27 and 27') run obliquely inferiorly and laterally and meet in the midline to form the **spinous process** (28) with its *two tubercles.*

Fig. 2

Fig. 3

Fig. 4

The atlanto-axial joints

The mechanical linkage between atlas and axis is achieved by **three mechanically linked joints:**
* *an axial joint*, i.e. the **median atlanto-axial joint**, with the dens axis serving as a pivot (see p. 197)
* *two symmetrical lateral joints*, i.e. the **lateral atlanto-axial joints** between the **inferior surfaces of the lateral masses of the atlas** and the **superior articular surfaces of the axis.**

Figure 5 (**axis seen in perspective**) and Figure 6 (lateral view) illustrate the shape and orientation of its **oval superior articular facet** (5); its great axis runs anteroposteriorly and it *is convex anteroposteriorly* along a *curve* represented by **xx′** but *straight transversely*. Thus its surface can be viewed as a section from **the surface of a cylinder** C with **axis Z** directed laterally and *slightly inferiorly* so that the articular facet faces superiorly and slightly laterally in the style of a 'shoulder strap' on a military uniform. The cylinder (*shown here as transparent*) from which these facets are cut comprises the lateral part of the axis and just overhangs the **distal tip of the transverse process.**

These two diagrams also reveal the rather unusual shape of the **dens**, which is roughly *cylindrical* but *bent posteriorly*. It bears:
* anteriorly a **shield-like articular facet** (1), which is slightly **biconvex** and *articulates with the articular facet* of the **anterior arch of the atlas**
* posteriorly a cartilage-lined **groove** (7), which is concave transversely and articulates with the functionally critical **transverse ligament** (see pp. 194 and 196)

A **parasagittal** section through the **lateral masses of the atlas** (Fig. 7) reveals the **orientations and curvatures** of the various articular surfaces:
* The curved outline of the **median atlanto-axial joint** with the **dens facet** (1) and the **articular facet of the anterior arch of the atlas** (2) is shown transected in the midsagittal plane; it lies on a circle with **centre of curvature Q** located behind the dens.
* The **superior facet of the lateral mass of the atlas** (3) is *convex anteroposteriorly* and *facing directly posteriorly*; it articulates with the *occipital condyle*.
* The **inferior facet of the lateral mass of the atlas** (4) is convex anteroposteriorly and lies on a circle with **centre of curvature O** and a radius *shorter than that of circle* **Q**.
* The **superior facet of the axis** (5) is convex anteroposteriorly and lies on a **circle with centre of curvature P** and a radius roughly equal to that of the circle with centre **O**. Thus the two articular surfaces (4 and 5) rest **on each other like two wheels.** The star indicates the centre of the movement of flexion-extension of the atlas on the axis (see Figs 9 and 10, p. 194).
* Finally, **the inferior facet of the axis** (6) *faces inferiorly and anteriorly*. It is almost flat, but its gently curved surface belongs to a *wide circle* with centre of curvature **R** lying inferiorly and posteriorly. It articulates with the *superior facet of the articular process of C3* (see p. 211).

Fig. 5

Fig. 6

Fig. 7

Flexion-extension in the lateral and median atlanto-axial joints

If the lateral masses of the atlas rolled without gliding on the superior articular surfaces of the axis during **flexion** (Fig. 8), then the **point of contact** between these two convex surfaces would move **anteriorly** and the line joining the centre of curvature P to the point of contact of these two surfaces would move from PA to PA′. At the same time, the joint space between the anterior arch of the atlas and the anterior facet of the dens should **gape** superiorly (b).

Likewise, if the lateral masses of the atlas rolled without gliding on the superior articular surfaces of the axis during **extension** (Fig. 9), their point of contact should **move** posteriorly, and the line joining the centre of curvature P to the contact point should move from PB to PB′. At the same time, the joint space between the anterior arch of the atlas and the anterior surface of the dens should **gape** inferiorly (b).

In real life a **careful scrutiny of lateral radiographs fails to show any gaping** (Fig. 10); this is due to the **transverse ligament** (T), which keeps the anterior arch of the atlas and the dens in close contact (see p. 196).

Therefore, the real centre of the movement of flexion-extension of the atlas on the axis (see Figure 7, p. 193) is neither P, the centre of curvature of the superior surface of the axis, nor Q, the centre of curvature of the anterior facet of the dens, but a **third point** (shown here as a red star) lying roughly in the centre of the dens seen from the side. As a result, during flexion-extension the inferior facets of the lateral masses of the atlas **roll and glide simultaneously** on the superior articular surfaces of the axis, just like the femoral condyles on the tibial articular surface.

It must be stressed, however, that the presence of a deformable structure, i.e. the transverse ligament, **forming the posterior wall of the median atlanto-axial joint**, allows some flexibility in the joint. The ligament, fitting tightly in a groove on the posterior surface of the dens, can bend *upwards during extension and downwards during flexion,* just like the chord of an arc. This also explains why the cavity of this joint is not entirely bony. The same reasoning also applies to the annular ligament of the superior radio-ulnar joint, which is also a pivot joint which is half osseous and half ligamentous (see Volume 1).

Thus the transverse ligament is **vitally important**, since it *keeps the atlas from gliding anteriorly on the axis.* Dislocation of this joint, often traumatic, can be **immediately lethal** as a result of compression of the medulla oblongata by the dens (Fig. 11). As the atlas is displaced anteriorly (red arrow), the dens literally rams (black arrow) into the neuraxis (light blue).

Fig. 8

Fig. 9

Fig. 11

Fig. 10

195

Rotation in the lateral and median atlanto-axial joints

We have just studied the median atlanto-axial joint from the side. **A superior view with the entire atlas included** (Fig. 12) and a **blown-up view** (Fig. 13) make it easy to understand its structure and its role in rotation. The **median atlanto-axial joint** is a **pivot joint** with two interlocked **pseudocylindrical surfaces:**

- The solid cylindrical surface, i.e. the **dens** (1), is not strictly cylindrical and therefore provides the joint with a second degree of freedom for **flexion-extension movements.** It has two **articular facets**, one on its anterior surface (4) and one on its posterior surface (11).
- The cavity receiving the solid cylinder (i.e. the **empty cylinder**) completely surrounds the dens and consists *anteriorly* of the **anterior arch of the atlas** (2) and *laterally* of the **lateral masses of the atlas.** Each lateral mass has on its medial surface a very distinct **tubercle** (7 and 7′) and gives attachment to a strong ligament running transversely behind the dens, i.e. the **transverse ligament of the atlas** (6).

The dens is thus encased within an **osteoligamentous ring** and makes contact with it at **two very different joints:**

- **anteriorly**, a **synovial joint** with an **articular cavity** (5), a **synovial capsule** and two recesses, one on the left (8) and one on the right (9); the joint surfaces are the **anterior facet of the dens** (4) and the **posterior facet of the anterior arch of the atlas** (3)
- **posteriorly**, a joint *without a capsule* and embedded within the *fibro-adipose tissue* (10), which fills the space between the osteoligamentous ring and the dens; the joint surfaces are **fibrocartilaginous**, the one **on the posterior surface of the dens** (11) and the other on the **anterior surface of the transverse ligament of the atlas** (12).

During rotation, for example to the left (Fig. 13), the dens (1) stays put while the osteoligamentous ring formed by the atlas and the transverse ligament **rotates anticlockwise** around a centre (white cross) lying on the axis of the dens, relaxing the capsular ligament on the left (9) and stretching it on the right (8). **At the same time, movement takes place in the mechanically linked right and left atlanto-axial joints.** During rotation from left to right (Fig. 14) the left lateral mass of the atlas moves forward (red arrow L-R), while the right lateral mass recedes. During rotation from right to left (Fig. 15) the converse occurs (blue arrow R-L).

The *superior articular surfaces of the axis* are, however, **convex anteroposteriorly** (Fig. 16). Therefore, the path taken by the lateral masses of the atlas is not straight in the horizontal plane but **convex superiorly** (Fig. 17), so that when the atlas rotates around its **vertical axis W**, its lateral masses travel from **x** to **x′** or from **y** to **y′**.

If only the circle corresponding to the **curvature of the inferior facet of each lateral mass of the atlas** (Fig. 16) is shown, it is clear that in the intermediate position or the position of zero rotation, the circle with centre **o** is **at its highest** location on the superior articular surface of the axis. When this circle moves anteriorly o′ it descends on the **anterior border of the superior surface of the axis** for a distance of 2-3 mm (e), while its centre descends for half this distance (e/2). The *same displacements occur when the circle moves posteriorly o′*.

When the atlas rotates on the axis it **drops vertically for a distance of 2–3 mm** in a **helical** movement, but the turns of helix are very tight. Furthermore, there are two helices with **opposite turns**: one for rotation to the right and the other for rotation to the left.

Fig. 12

Fig. 13

L-R

R-L

Fig. 14

Fig. 15

Fig. 16

Fig. 17

The articular surfaces of the atlanto-occipital joint

There are in fact **two mechanically linked and symmetrical atlanto-occipital** joints formed by the **superior articular surfaces of the lateral masses of the atlas** and the **articular surfaces of the occipital condyles**.

In a superior view of the atlas (Fig. 18) its articular surfaces appear **oval, with their main axes running obliquely anteriorly and medially** and converging at a point N on the midline and slightly anterior to the anterior arch of the atlas. Occasionally they are waisted in the middle and may even be divided into two separate facets. They are lined with cartilage and are **biconcave with roughly similar curvatures**. Therefore these surfaces can be considered as **parts of the surface of a sphere** (Fig. 19) with **centre O** located above the articular surfaces and vertically above Q, which is the point of intersection of the axis of symmetry of the atlas and the line joining the posterior borders of the two articular facets. **Q** is also the **centre of curvature of the articular surfaces in the horizontal plane; P** is **their centre of curvature in the vertical plane**. The sphere (considered transparent) is seen (green dashes) resting very precisely on the superior articular surfaces of the lateral masses of the atlas.

A posterior view of the atlanto-occipital joints (Fig. 20) confirms that the surfaces of the occipital condyles also lie on the surface of the same sphere, whose **centre O** lies within the cranium *above the foramen magnum*. Thus the atlanto-occipital joint can be considered as equivalent to an **enarthrosis**, i.e. a joint with spherical articular surfaces (Fig. 19) with **three axes** and three movements:

- **axial rotation** around a vertical axis **QO**
- **flexion-extension** around a transverse axis **zz'** passing through **O**
- **lateral** flexion **around** an anteroposterior axis **PO**

of even smaller ranges.

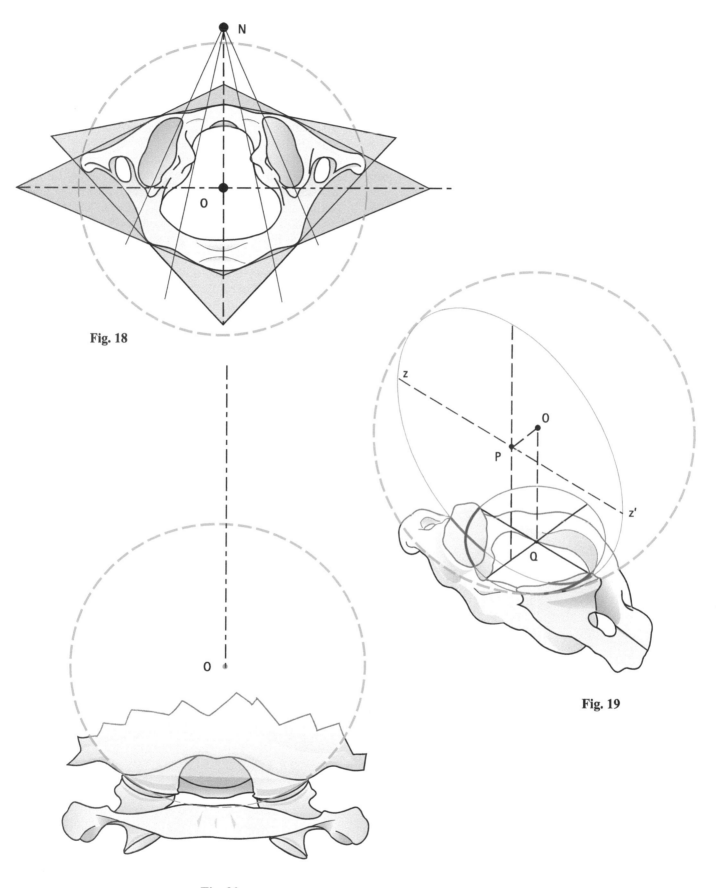

Fig. 18

Fig. 19

Fig. 20

Rotation in the atlanto-occipital joints

When the **occiput rotates on the atlas** (Fig. 21), its rotation is part of the general rotation of the atlas on the axis about a vertical axis passing through the centre of the dens. This rotation, however, is not a simple process, since it actively **stretches some ligaments**, in particular the **alar ligament** (L, green arrow). This diagram, representing a coronal cut taken vertically through the occipital bone (A) and the **lateral masses of the atlas** (B), shows *rotation to the left* of the occipital condyle on the atlas, which is observed as an *anterior gliding movement of the right occipital condyle on the right lateral mass of the atlas* (red arrow 1). But at the same time, the **alar ligament** (L) **wraps itself** around the dens and **is stretched, pulling the right occipital condyle to the left** (white arrow 2).

Therefore, rotation to the left (blue arrow) is associated at once with a **2-3 mm translation to the left** and **a lateral flexion of the occiput** to the right (red arrow). As a result, there is no pure rotation at the atlanto-occipital joint but a rotation associated with a **translation and a flexion**.

Now in kinematics a **rotation associated with a translation is equivalent to another rotation** with similar range but with a different centre of rotation, which is easy to represent diagrammatically. **A superior view** (Fig. 22) shows the atlas in light colour, the axis (seen through the foramen magnum) in darker colour and, on top of the **lateral articular facets of the atlas** (at) the facets of the occipital condyles (oc), shown as transparent. During rotation to the left over an angle (**a**) around the **centre of the dens** (D), the occiput is displaced laterally to the left for 2-3 mm in the direction of the **vector V**. It is now easy to locate the real centre of rotation in a **point P** lying slightly to the left of the plane of symmetry and on the line **z** *joining the posterior borders of the lateral masses of the atlas*. Therefore, the **real centre** of rotation at the atlanto-occipital joint moves between two extreme points, **P** for rotation to the left and **P′** for rotation to the right. This process causes the real centre of rotation O to recede towards the centre of the foramen magnum so that the real axis of its normally elliptical rotation coincides with the anatomical axis of the medulla oblongata – *the ideal position for torsion of the neuraxis.*

Fig. 21

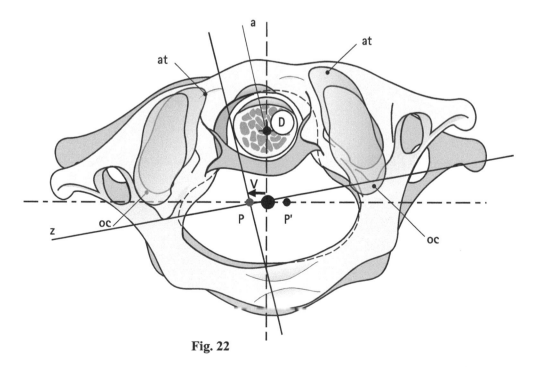

Fig. 22

Lateral flexion and flexion-extension in the atlanto-occipital joint

A coronal section taken vertically through the occipital bone, the atlas and C3 (Fig. 23) shows that during **lateral flexion** there is **no movement in the atlanto-axial joint.** Lateral flexion occurs **only between the axis and C3** on the one hand, and between the **occipital bone and the atlas** on the other. Between the occipital bone and the atlas the range of movement is **small** and consists only of the **gliding of the occipital condyles** to the right for left lateral flexion and vice versa. In Figure 23, showing lateral flexion to the left, the left occipital condyle is seen **moving closer to the dens** without coming into contact with it because **the movement is checked by the tension developed in the capsular ligament of the atlanto-occipital joint,** especially by **the right alar ligament.** The **total range of lateral flexion** between the occipital bone and C3 is 8°, with 5° between the axis and C3 and 3° between the atlas and the occipital bone. **During flexion-extension of the occipital bone on the atlas** the occipital condyles glide on the lateral masses of the atlas. **During flexion** (Fig. 24) the occipital condyles recede on the lateral masses of the atlas while the **squama of the occipital bone moves away** from the posterior arch of the atlas (red arrow).

As the latter movement is always associated with **flexion in the atlanto-axial joint, the posterior arches of the atlas and of the axis move apart** (red arrow), and the anterior arch of the atlas glides downwards on the anterior facet of the dens (red arrow). Flexion is checked by the **tension developed in the capsular and posterior ligaments** (the posterior atlanto-occipital membrane and ligamentum nuchae).

During extension (Fig. 25) the occipital condyles glide anteriorly on the lateral masses of the atlas. At the same time, the occipital bone **moves towards the posterior arch of the atlas** (blue arrow) and, as the **atlanto-axial joint is also extended,** the **posterior arches of the atlas and of the axis approach each other** (blue arrow), while the anterior arch of the atlas **glides upwards** on the anterior facet of the dens (blue arrow). Extension is checked by the **impact of these three bones. During violent movements of forced extension** the posterior arch of the atlas is caught as if in a nutcracker **between the occipital bone and the posterior arch of the axis** and **can be fractured.** The total range of **flexion-extension is 15°** at the **atlanto-occipital joint.**

Fig. 23

Flexion

15°

Fig. 24

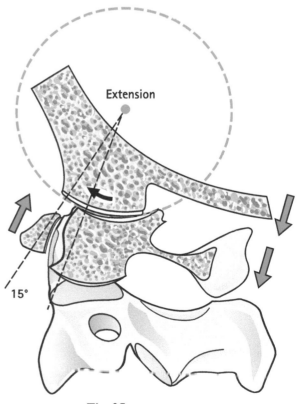

Extension

15°

Fig. 25

The suboccipital ligaments of the spine

The very numerous and very strong ligaments of the suboccipital spine can be seen in a sagittal view (Fig. 26), where the neuraxis is shown as transparent, i.e. the brainstem and the medulla as B and the spinal cord as C. The legends are the same in Figures 26 to 34 inclusive.

First the **bony structures** are shown in cross-section from above downwards:

- the **basilar process** (a) and the **squama** (b) of the occipital bone
- the anterior (e) and posterior (f) arches of the atlas
- the **dens** (g) and the axis (k) (sagittal views)
- the anterior articular facet (h) of the dens in contact with the posterior articular facet (i) of the anterior arch of the atlas
- the rest of the **axis** featuring its spinous process (n) and a section of its left lamina (o)
- below the axis, the body (q), spinous process (s) and left lamina (r) of C3
- the posterior cranial fossa (seen in perspective) containing the cerebellum, the brainstem and the beginning of the medulla oblongata B above the **foramen magnum.**

Next are shown the ligaments:

- the **apical ligament of dens** (1), short and thick, running vertically between the basilar process of the occipital bone and the apex of the dens
- the **transverse ligament** (3, seen in cross-section) in contact with the posterior articular facet of the dens
- the **transverso-occipital ligament** (4) between the superior margin of the transverse ligament and the basilar process of the occipital bone
- the **transverso-axial ligament** (5) between the inferior margin of the transverse ligament and the posterior surface of the body of the axis (these last three ligaments form the **cruciate ligament,** see Fig. 29)
- the **median occipito-axial ligament** (7), behind the cruciate ligament, runs from the basilar process to the posterior surface of the body of the axis and is continuous posteriorly with the **lateral occipito-axial ligaments** (not shown here)
- the **capsule** of the atlanto-occipital joint (9)
- the **posterior longitudinal ligament** (12), lying behind the median and lateral occipito-axial ligaments, is inserted into the groove in the basilar process and the inferior border of the axis; it spans the *full length of the spine down to the sacral canal*

- the **anterior atlanto-occipital membrane**, lying anterior to the apical ligament of dens, is made up of a deep (13) and of a superficial (14) band and runs from the basilar process to the anterior arch of the atlas
- the **anterior atlanto-axial ligament** (16) is a downward prolongation of the anterior atlanto-occipital ligament and runs from the inferior border of the arch of the atlas to the body of the axis. Anterior to the dens and to the apical ligament of dens, and posterior to the median atlanto-occipital and atlanto-axial ligaments, there is a fibro-adipose space which contains the median atlanto-axial joint and its capsule (17)
- the **anterior longitudinal ligament** (18) overlies all these ligaments anteriorly. It arises from the basilar process, bridges over the anterior arch of the atlas and is inserted into the body of the axis (18′). From there it extends along the anterior surfaces of the vertebrae right down to the sacrum and is attached to the anterior borders of the intervertebral discs (d) and the vertebral bodies (v).

The posterior arches are linked by the following ligaments:

- the **posterior atlanto-occipital ligament** (19), running from the posterior margin of the foramen magnum to the posterior arch of the atlas, is the equivalent of a **ligamentum flavum** 19′; it is pierced (C1) on each side just behind the lateral mass of the atlas by the *ascending occipital artery* and *the exiting first cervical nerve*
- the **posterior atlanto-axial ligament** (21), connecting the posterior arches of the atlas to the axis *like a ligamentum flavum,* is pierced (C2) behind the atlanto-axial joint by the exiting *second cervical nerve*
- the **interspinous ligament** (22), which unites the posterior arch of the atlas and the spinous process of the axis, interconnects the spinous processes of the cervical vertebrae below
- the **ligamentum nuchae** (23), a very thick, fibrous septum homologous to a supraspinous ligament, is attached to the midline of the occipital bone and separates the nuchal muscles into two compartments, a right and a left
- the **capsule** of the facet joint (24) between the axis and C3 bounds posteriorly the intervertebral foramen (C3) containing the third cervical nerve
- the **ligamentum flavum** (25) unites the posterior arches of the axis and C3.

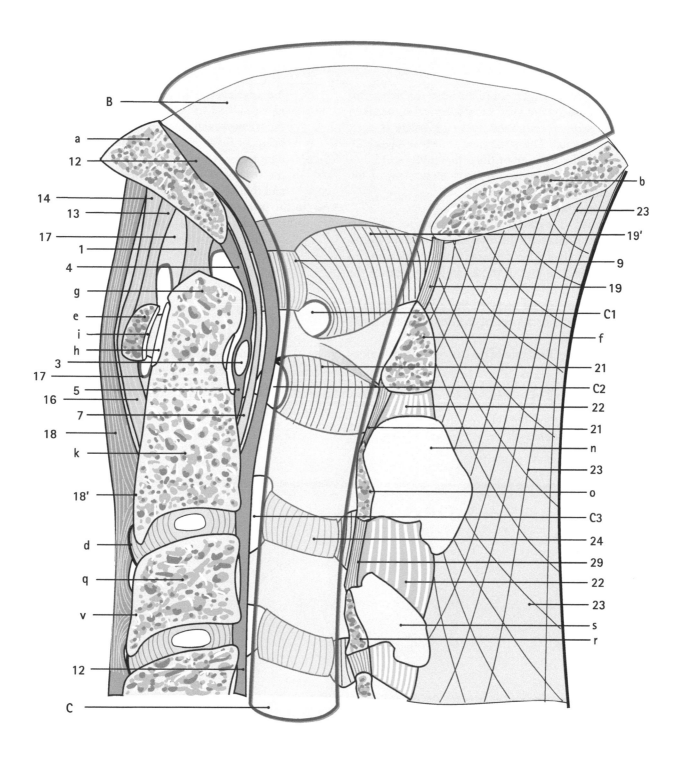

Fig. 26

The suboccipital ligaments

Figure 27 illustrates the arrangement of the posterior suboccipital ligaments; it is a **posterior view** of the cervical spine taken in a *verticofrontal plane through the posterior arches* (f, t, r), which have been resected. The structures shown in Figure 26 are still visible, with the addition of the following:

- the intracranial surface (a) and a cross-section (b) of the occipital squama
- the **occipital condyles** (c)
- the **lateral masses of the atlas** (d) and its anterior arch (e)
- the **atlanto-axial joints** with the inferior facets of the lateral masses of the atlas (l) and the superior facets of the axis (m)
- a section of the pedicle and of the articular process of the axis (t)
- the posterior surface of the body of the axis, the articular facet (h) on the posterior aspect of the dens and the transverse ligament
- the posterior surface of the body of C3 (q) with cross-sections of its laminae (r).

The following ligaments are attached to the various bones:
- **in the deep plane** (Fig. 28):
  - the apical ligament of dens (1)
  - the **two alar ligaments** (2)
  - the **transverse ligament** (3), running horizontally between the two lateral masses of the atlas
  - the **transverso-occipital ligament** (4), which has been cut flush at the posterior margin of the transverse ligament
  - the **transverso-axial ligament** (5), similarly resected and folded downwards
- **in the intermediate plane** (Fig. 29):
  - the intact **cruciate ligament** (6), made up of the transverse, the transverso-occipital and the transverso-axial ligaments
  - laterally, the capsular ligament of the **atlanto-occipital joint** (9), reinforced laterally by the **alar ligament** (10) above and the capsule of the atlanto-axial joint (11) below
- **in the superficial plane** (Fig. 30):
  - the **median occipito-axial ligament** (7) directly continuous with the alar ligaments (8) laterally and the partially resected **posterior longitudinal ligament** (12) axially.

Fig. 27

Fig. 28

Fig. 29

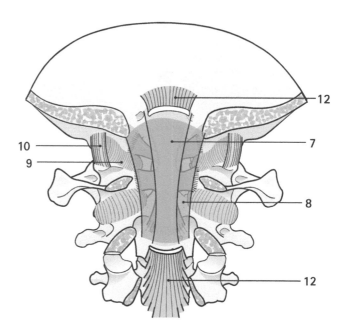

Fig. 30

The suboccipital ligaments (continued)

Figures 31 and 33 show only the bony structures, whereas Figures 32 and 34 also show the attached ligaments.

Figure 31 (anterior) illustrates all the bony structures already mentioned. Figure 32 contains the **anterior ligaments** as follows:

- the **anterior atlanto-occipital membrane**, with its deep (13) and superficial (14) layers, the latter partially overlying the capsule of the atlanto-occipital joint (9)
- the **anterolateral atlanto-occipital membrane** (15) lying anterior to the former and running obliquely from the basilar process of the occipital bone to the transverse process of the atlas
- the **anterior atlanto-axial ligament** (16), continuous laterally with the capsule of the atlanto-axial joint (11)
- the **anterior longitudinal ligament** (18), shown only in its left half
- the **capsular ligament** of the joint between the axis and C3 (23).

A posterior view of the bony structures (Fig. 33) shows the posterior arches of the atlas, of the axis and of the third vertebra, with the spinal canal visible between the vertebrae and the foramen magnum between the atlas and the occipital squama.

A posterior view of the ligaments (Fig. 34) shows on the **right side** the ligaments covering the anterior surfaces of the spinal canal (already illustrated in Fig. 29):

- the alar (7) and the lateral occipito-axial (8) ligaments
- the **capsular ligament** of the atlanto-occipital joint (9), reinforced by the **lateral atlanto-occipital ligament** (10)
- also seen is the **vertebral artery** as it runs upwards through the foramina transversaria and bends posteriorly and then medially to skirt the posterior border of the lateral mass of the atlas (25).

On the left side the posterior ligaments include the following:

- the **posterior atlanto-occipital membrane** (19), covered by the atlanto-occipital ligament (20), and extending from the occipital squama to the transverse process of the atlas
- **the posterior atlanto-axial ligament** (21)
- the **interspinous ligaments** (22) covered by the ligamentum nuchae (only their left halves are shown here)
- finally, the **capsular ligament** of the joint between the axis and C3 (24).

The following are also visible in Figure 34:

- the **first cervical nerve** (26) emerging from the foramen for the vertebral artery
- the **second cervical nerve** (27), whose posterior ramus gives off the greater occipital nerve
- the **posterior ramus of the third cervical nerve** (28) exiting through the intervertebral foramen, i.e. in front of the joint between the axis and C3 (24).

Fig. 31

Fig. 32

Fig. 33

Fig. 34

The structure of a typical cervical vertebra

A **posterosuperior view** (Fig. 35) of a typical cervical vertebra illustrates its various components (which are also shown 'disassembled' in Fig. 36) as follows:

- The **vertebral body** (1) with its **superior discal surface** (2) is raised on both sides by two transversely flat buttresses, i.e. the uncinate processes (3 and 3′), which enclose the **articular surfaces** for the inferior discal surface of the overlying vertebra.
- Also seen are the **flat area** (4) on the anterior margin of the superior discal surface and the beak-like antero-inferior prolongation (5) of the anterior margin of the inferior discal surface.

As a whole, the superior discal surface is *concave transversely and convex anteroposteriorly* just like a **saddle.** With the help of the intervertebral disc (not shown) it articulates with the reciprocally shaped inferior discal surface of the overlying vertebra. This articular complex is similar to a saddle joint and allows flexion-extension to occur preferentially, since lateral flexion is restricted by the uncinate processes, which guide the anteroposterior movements during flexion-extension.

- To the posterior part of the lateral surface of the vertebral body are attached the **pedicles** (6 and 6′), which give origin to the posterior arches and the **anterior roots of the transverse processes** (7 and 7′).

The cervical transverse processes are unusual in their shape and orientation (Fig. 37): they are hollowed into a superiorly concave *groove*, and they are directed anteriorly and laterally, forming an angle of 60° with the sagittal plane. However, they slope slightly obliquely downwards at an angle of 15°. The posteromedial extremity of the groove lines the intervertebral foramen, and its anterolateral extremity is flanked by **two tubercles**, which give attachment to the scalene muscles. The groove is perforated by the **foramen transversarium**, through which ascends the **vertebral artery.** The **cervical nerve**, leaving the vertebral canal at the intervertebral foramen, runs along this groove and crosses the vertebral artery at right angles before emerging between the two tubercles of the transverse process.

- This foramen in the groove of the transverse process gives the impression that the process arises by **two roots**, i.e. one attached directly to the vertebral body and the other to the articular process.
- The **articular processes** (9 and 9′) lie posterior and lateral to the body, to which they are connected by the **pedicles** (6 and 6′). They bear the **articular facets**; only the superior facets (10 and 10′), which articulate with the inferior facets of the overlying vertebra, are shown here.
- The **posterior arch** is completed by the **laminae** (11 and 11′), which meet in the midline to form the bifid **spinous process** (12).
- The **posterior arch** is thus made up successively of the pedicles, the articular processes, the laminae and the spinous processes.
- The **intervertebral foramen** is bounded inferiorly by the pedicle, medially by the vertebral body and the uncinate process, and laterally by the articular process.
- The **vertebral canal** (C) is triangular in shape and is bounded anteriorly by the vertebral body and posteriorly by the vertebral arch.

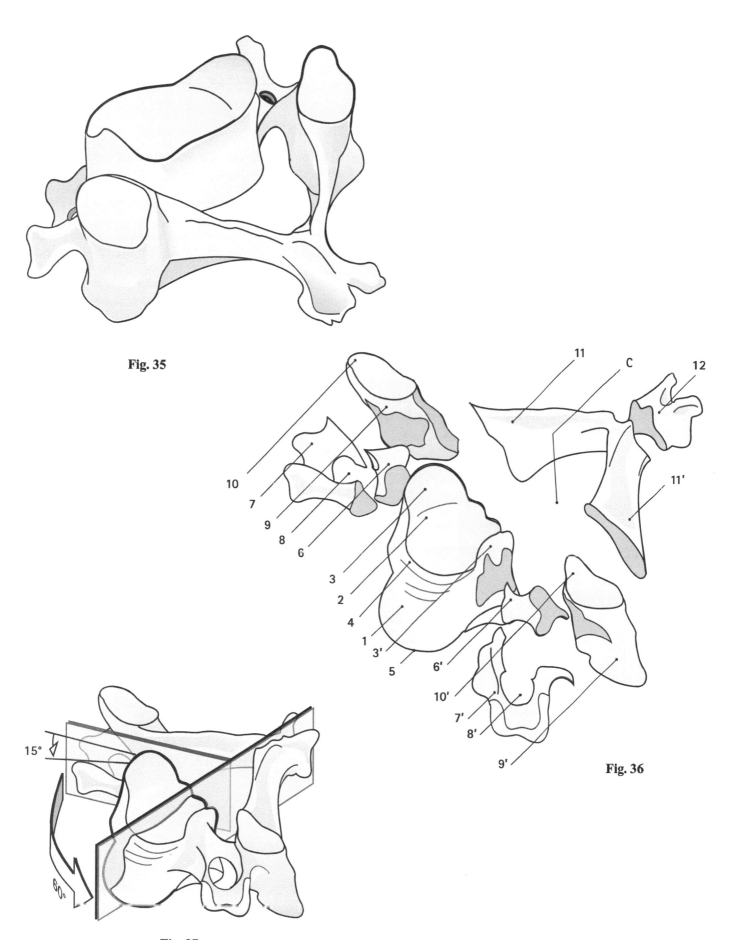

Fig. 35

Fig. 36

Fig. 37

15°

60°

The ligaments of the lower cervical spine

The very unusual intervertebral ligaments in the suboccipital region have already been presented. Some of them extend down into the lower cervical region. The lower cervical intervertebral ligaments can be seen in detail **on a section taken in perspective from behind and from the left side** (Fig. 38) and revealing a cervical vertebra cut sagittally with its **superior discal surface** (a) and its raised uncinate process (b). This vertebra is united to the underlying vertebra by the **intervertebral disc** with its clearly visible components, i.e. the annulus fibrosus (1) and the nucleus pulposus (2).

The **anterior longitudinal ligament** (3) and the **posterior longitudinal ligament** (4) lie respectively anterior and posterior to the vertebral body. On each side the **uncovertebral joint** is bounded by a capsule (5).

The **facet joints** are formed by articular facets (d) united by a capsule (6), which is also shown opened (6'). Between the **laminae** on both sides run the ligamenta flava (7), one of which is shown after transection (7').

The **spinous processes** (j) are interconnected by the interspinous ligaments (8) continuous posteriorly with the supraspinous ligament, which is well defined in the cervical region as the **ligamentum nuchae** (9) and gives attachment on its two surfaces to the **trapezius** and the **splenius.**

The **transverse processes** with their anterior (e) and posterior (f) tubercles are interconnected by the **intertransverse ligaments** (10).

Also visible at the level of the transverse process are the **foramen transversarium** (g) and the intervertebral foramina (i), which are bounded as follows:

- superiorly by the **vertebral pedicle** (h)
- posteriorly and laterally by the **articular processes** and the **facet joint**
- anteriorly and medially by the **vertebral body**, the **intervertebral disc** consisting of the annulus fibrosus (1), the nucleus pulposus (2) and the **uncinate process** (b).

Fig. 38

Flexion-extension in the lower cervical spine

In the neutral position the vertebral bodies (Fig. 39, **lateral view**) are united by an intervertebral disc, whose nucleus pulposus is stable and whose annulus fibrosus is evenly stretched. The **cervical vertebrae** (Fig. 40) are also connected by their articular processes, whose facets are oblique inferiorly and posteriorly. In the lower cervical spine these facets are slightly concave anteriorly in the parasagittal plane, with their centres of curvature lying quite far inferiorly and anteriorly. As a result of the cervical lordosis, these centres of curvature are set farther apart than the planes of the articular surfaces themselves. On page 218 the significance of the convergence of these axes will become apparent. **During extension** the body of the upper vertebra (Fig. 41) tilts and glides **posteriorly**, the intervertebral space becomes narrower posteriorly than anteriorly, the nucleus is driven slightly anteriorly and the anterior fibres of the annulus are stretched further. Since this posterior gliding of the vertebral body does not occur around the centres of curvature of the articular facets, the interspace of the facet joints (Fig. 42) **gapes** anteriorly. In fact, the superior facet not only glides inferiorly and posteriorly relative to the inferior facet, it also forms with it an angle x', which is equal to the angle of extension x and to the angle x'' between the two **normals** (red) to these articular facets. Extension (blue arrow E) is checked by the **tension developed in the anterior longitudinal ligament** and especially by **bony contact**, i.e. the impact of the superior articular process of the lower vertebra on the transverse process of the upper vertebra, and especially the **impact of one posterior arch on the other** via their ligaments.

During flexion the body of the upper vertebra (Fig. 43) tilts and glides **anteriorly**, compressing the intervertebral disc anteriorly, chasing the nucleus posteriorly and stretching the posterior fibres of the annulus. This anterior tilting of the upper vertebra is helped by the flat area in the superior surface of the lower vertebra, which allows the beak-like projection of the inferior surface of the upper vertebra to move past.

Just as with extension, flexion of the upper vertebra (Fig. 44) does not occur around the centres of curvature of the articular facets. As a result, the inferior facet of the upper vertebra moves superiorly and anteriorly, while the joint space between these facets is opened out inferiorly and posteriorly by an angle y', which is equal to the angle of flexion y and to the angle y'' between the two **normals** (red) to the articular facets.

Flexion (red arrow F) is not checked by bony impact but **only by the tension developed in the posterior longitudinal ligament**, the capsular ligaments of the facet joints, the ligamenta flava, the interspinous ligaments and the ligamentum nuchae (the cervical supraspinous ligament).

During car accidents with **impact from behind** or from in front, the cervical spine is often very strongly extended and then flexed. This produces the **whiplash injury**, related to stretching or even tearing of the various ligaments, and in extreme cases **to anterior dislocation of the articular processes.** The inferior articular processes of the upper vertebra become hooked onto the anterosuperior margins of the articular processes of the lower vertebra. This type of dislocation, including this hooking process, is very difficult to reduce and endangers the medulla oblongata and the cervical cord with the **risk of sudden death, quadriplegia or paraplegia.** This underscores the need for caution in the handling of people with this type of injury.

Fig. 39

Fig. 40

Fig. 41

Fig. 42

Fig. 43

Fig. 44

The movements at the uncovertebral joints

In addition to the movements at the facet joints and at the intervertebral discs there are in the cervical region movements taking place at two additional small articular processes, i.e. **at the uncovertebral joints.**

A **coronal section** (Fig. 45) shows two vertebral discal surfaces and the disc with its nucleus and its annulus, but the disc does not reach the edge of the vertebra. In fact the superior surface is raised laterally by two buttresses lying in a sagittal plane. Each uncinate process has its cartilaginous articular surface facing **upwards and inwards** and articulates with the inferolateral border of the upper vertebra, via a semilunate cartilaginous articular surface facing **downwards and outwards.** This small joint is enclosed in a **capsule** blending with the intervertebral disc: it is therefore a **synovial joint.** During **flexion-extension**, when the body of the upper vertebra glides anteriorly or posteriorly, the articular facets of the uncovertebral joints **also glide relative** to each other. The uncinate processes guide the vertebral body during this movement.

During lateral flexion (Fig. 46) the interspaces of these uncovertebral joints gape by an angle **a′** or **a″**, equal to the angle of lateral flexion **a** and to the angle between the two horizontal lines **nn′** and **mm′** joining the transverse processes. The diagram also shows the **contralateral** displacement of the nucleus and stretching of the capsular ligament of the ipsilateral uncovertebral joint.

In real life the movements of the uncovertebral joints are far more complex. We shall see later (p. 218) that pure lateral flexion does not occur but is **always associated with rotation and extension.** Therefore, during these movements, the interspace of the uncovertebral joint gapes not only superiorly or inferiorly but also anteriorly as the upper vertebra moves backwards. The diagrams (Figs 47 and 48, seen in perspective with extremely simplified vertebrae) are meant to explain how these movements take place. It would be a good idea to come back to these diagrams after mastering the mechanism of combined lateral flexion-rotation.

Fig. 45

Fig. 46

Fig. 47

Fig. 48

Orientation of the articular facets: the composite axis of lateral flexion-rotation

Lateral flexion and rotation in the lower cervical spine are governed by the *orientation of the articular facets* of the articular processes, which precludes any pure rotation or pure lateral flexion.

Figure 49 shows that the superior articular facets of a midzone cervical vertebra, e.g. the **fifth cervical vertebra** (C5), are flat and lie within the same plane **P**, oblique, inferiorly and posteriorly. Therefore, any gliding of the overlying vertebra (C4) can only be of two types:

- a **global gliding movement upwards**, i.e. equivalent to **flexion** or a global gliding movement downwards, equivalent to **extension**
- a **differential gliding movement** with the left facet of C4 moving upwards and forwards (arrow a) while the right facet moves downwards and backwards (arrow b). This differential gliding in the plane **P** is therefore tantamount to a rotation around an axis **A** perpendicular to plane **P** and lying in the sagittal plane. The rotation of C4 around the inferiorly and anteriorly oblique axis **A** imparts to it a combined movement of rotation-lateral flexion, which depends on the obliquity of axis **A.**

Horizontal sections taken through the facet joints show that the superior and inferior surfaces of these facets are not strictly flat but are:

- **slightly convex posteriorly** for C6 and C7 (Fig. 50)
- **slightly concave anteriorly** for C3 and C4 (Fig. 51).

These observations do not contradict the previous statements, since the plane **P** (Fig. 49) can be replaced by a wide spherical surface whose centre of curvature would lie on the axis **A** below the vertebra **A'** for C6 and C7 (Fig. 52) and above the vertebra **A″** for C3 and C4 (Fig. 53). Thus the composite axis of lateral flexion-extension still coincides with the axis **A** of Figure 49

A lateral radiograph of the cervical spine (Fig. 54) illustrates the direction of the planes of the **articular facets** as follows:

- The planes **a to f** are all oblique relative to the vertical.
- Moreover, their obliquity increases caudocranially. Thus the plane **f**, corresponding to the interspace between C7 and T1, forms an angle of only 10° with the horizontal, whereas the plane **a**, corresponding to the interspace between C2 and C3, forms an angle of 40-45° with the horizontal. Therefore, there is an angle of 30-35° between the planes of the lowest (f) and of the highest (a) interspaces.

These planes, however, do not exactly converge at the same point. The obliquity of these planes fails to increase regularly caudocranially, with the last three planes (d-f) almost parallel, and the first three planes (a-c) which are by and large strongly convergent.

If a median is drawn at the level of each articular facet, the obliquity of the axes 1-6 increases regularly and fits within an angle of 30-35°, but importantly the lower axis 6 is nearly vertical, indicating an almost pure rotation at this level, whereas the highest axis 1 forms an angle of 40-45° with the vertical, indicating almost equal rotation and lateral flexion at this level.

Figure 54 (**diagram inspired by Penning**) also contains small black crosses indicating the centres of rotation and corresponding to the location of the transverse axis of flexion-extension of each upper vertebra. In the craniocaudal direction these centres of motion shift progressively more upwards and forwards in the vertebral body. The positions of these centres do not coincide with the theoretical centres (shown as small black stars) obtained from lateral radiographs taken in extreme positions of flexion and extension.

The main message is that the axis 1 to 6 of lateral flexion-rotation are **convergent**.

Fig. 51

Fig. 50

Fig. 49

Fig. 54

Fig. 52

Fig. 53

Combined lateral flexion-rotation in the lower cervical spine

The obliquity of the axis at each level of the spine accounts for the combined movement of **lateral flexion** and **rotation**, which is added to the movements of **flexion-extension. Along the whole length of the lower cervical spine** between C2 and T1 (Fig. 55, diagrammatic representation in space of the lower central cervical spine) there is an additional component of extension. In fact, at the level of T1, which lies along the spinal axis, movement between C7 and T1 leads to combined lateral flexion-rotation of C7, whereas movement between C6 and C7, which already starts in a position of lateral flexion-rotation, will lead this time not only to combined rotation-lateral flexion but also to an additional **movement of extension.** This combination of movements becomes more pronounced caudocranially. If this composite movement of the lower cervical spine is resolved along the three planes of reference with the use of anterior and lateral radiographs (unfortunately transverse radiographs cannot be taken, but CT scans can now be done), then the following three components can be observed:

- in the coronal plane (C) a component of lateral flexion (L)
- in the sagittal plane (S) a component of extension (E)
- in the transverse or horizontal plane (T) a component of rotation (R).

Therefore, apart from flexion-extension, the cervical spine can only perform **stereotypical** movements of mixed lateral flexion-rotation-extension, with extension being automatically offset in part by flexion in the lower cervical spine itself. Conversely, as we shall see (p. 228), the other unwanted components can only be offset in the upper cervical spine.

Fig. 56

Fig. 55

221

Geometric illustration of the movement of lateral flexion-rotation

The **movement of lateral flexion-extension can be illustrated geometrically** (Fig. 57) by simply using a three-dimensional diagram featuring the plane R of lateral flexion-rotation occurring about an axis **u.** This plane R corresponds to the previously defined plane shared by the articular facets. Since axis u is oblique, the plane R is also oblique at an angle **a** relative to the coronal (C) and transverse or horizontal (T) planes of reference. The sagittal plane S, perpendicular to the other two, contains the segment **k** (in red), which corresponds to the axis of symmetry of the upper vertebra as it rotates around the axis **u.**

This segment rotates to the right in the plane R around its axis (u) over an angle **b**, which is projected onto the transverse plane T as angle **c**. Its final position (l) then lies in the vertical plane P, which has simultaneously turned around the vertical line passing through **o.** In this new position the segment l is projected to l′ in the plane C. Likewise, in the plane T, this rotation is measured as the angle **c** at o″ between planes S and P. These projections represent:

- the component of **lateral flexion** in the plane C
- the component of **rotation** in the plane T.

When the upper vertebra rotates around the axis u it shifts the axis of rotation of the underlying vertebra to u′ while the next upper vertebra shifts its axis to u″. This explains how a new component of extension is generated, which can be calculated with the use of trigonometry. We shall not try to do so here.

The diagram (Fig. 58, in perspective) includes two cervical vertebrae one on top of the other and displays the right rotation (red arrow) of the upper vertebra around the axis u, while its left lateral masses move forwards and its right lateral masses recede. This rotation is represented by the dashed lines passing through the superior articular surfaces of each vertebra.

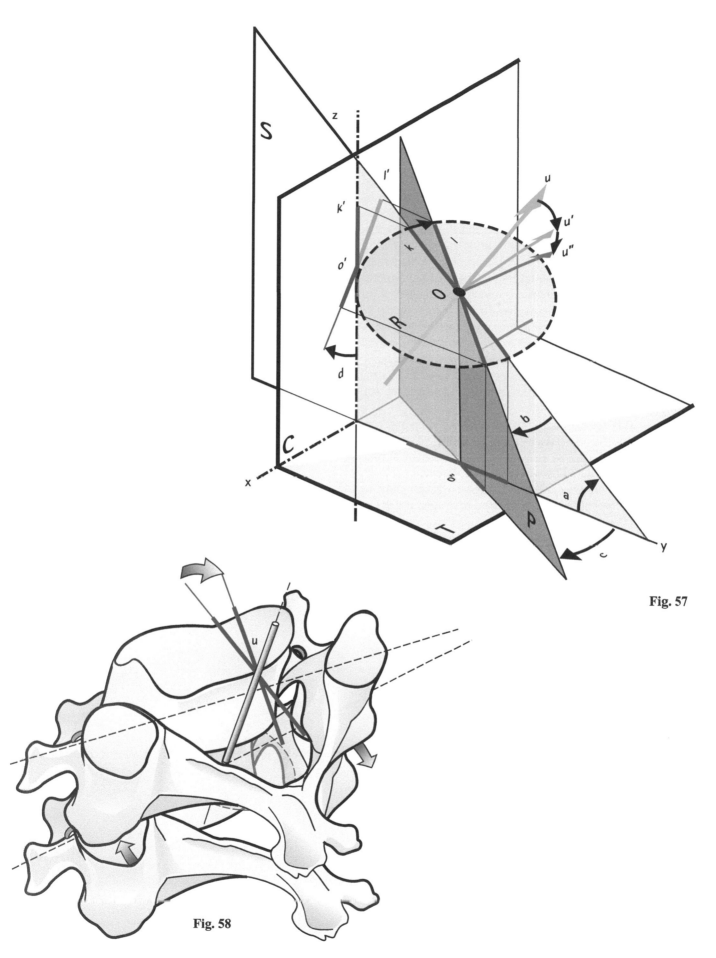

Fig. 57

Fig. 58

Mechanical model of the cervical spine

From a knowledge of the structural ideas already presented, and of the functional separation of the upper suboccipital and lower segments of the cervical spine, we have devised a **mechanical model** (Fig. 59) that illustrates the various modes of action of the joints in the cervical spine.

For the lower cervical spine between C2 and T1, only the composite movements of lateral flexion-rotation are shown taking place around oblique axes (see p. 226) in accordance with their anatomical obliquity and orientation relative to the vertebral bodies, which in this model are not connected by intervertebral discs. The vertebral bodies themselves limit the movements of lateral flexion-rotation. *We have deliberately omitted the movements of flexion-extension in order to bring out those of lateral flexion-rotation.*

The **suboccipital cervical spine** has been built in strict accordance with its mechanical properties, and it comprises the following:

- **a vertical axis** corresponding to the dens and allowing rotation and some flexion-extension of the elliptical end-plate representing the atlas, as a result of some mechanical play deliberately introduced between the end-plate and C2
- **an articular complex** of small range corresponding to the atlanto-occipital joint. It has **three orthogonal axes** as follows:
  - **a vertical axis** sited in the centre of the atlas end-plate
  - **two axes** perpendicular to each other and to the vertical axis. They represent the two axes of a *universal joint* corresponding to the axes of lateral flexion-rotation and flexion-extension at the atlanto-occipital joint.

The full details are clearly illustrated in Figure 64 on page 231. Globally the suboccipital spine is the equivalent of **an articular complex with three axes and three degrees of freedom**, connecting C2 to the occipital bone, which is shown in this model as a horizontal plank containing the three main reference planes of the head:

- the sagittal plane in **light grey**
- the coronal plane in **white**
- the transverse plane represented by a **grey-tinted plank** lying below the other two.

This model allows one to understand how the two segments of the cervical spine are *functionally complementary* and how *lateral flexion-right rotation of the lower segment is changed into pure lateral flexion* in the suboccipital segment by the loss of unwanted components due to a **contralateral rotation and a small flexion.**

By cutting out and folding the **simplified mechanical model** provided at the end of the book (see p. 327-330) the reader will be able to verify these observations.

Fig. 59

Movements of lateral flexion-rotation in the mechanical model

In this detailed view of the lower cervical spine (Fig. 60) each vertebra corresponds functionally to a posterior arch represented by a small plank lying obliquely downwards and backwards and supported by a wedge-shaped block. If we compare Figure 60 and Figure 54 (p. 219), it is obvious that the role of these wedge-shaped blocks is to reproduce the convergence of the planes of the articular surfaces and thus to reproduce the **cervical lordosis.**

The oblique axis of each vertebra is *shown here by an imperfectly tight screw*, which passes at right angles to the corresponding articular surface and provides linkage for the upper vertebra. Thus the upper vertebra can only move relative to the lower vertebra by rotation about this oblique axis (see Fig. 54).

If this model is rotated successively around its six axes, it will show a lateral flexion combined with a 50° range of **rotation** (Fig. 61), corresponding to that of the lower cervical spine, as well as a small component of extension not easily seen in these diagrams.

Also worth noting is the cylindrical shape of the upper surface of C2, which functionally represents the atlanto-axial joint (see Fig. 64, p. 231):

- it is **convex** anteroposteriorly, corresponds to the superior articular facets of the axis and allows movements of flexion-extension of the atlas to occur (not shown here)
- its **vertical axis** juts out and functionally represents the dens, which allows movements of rotation to take place.

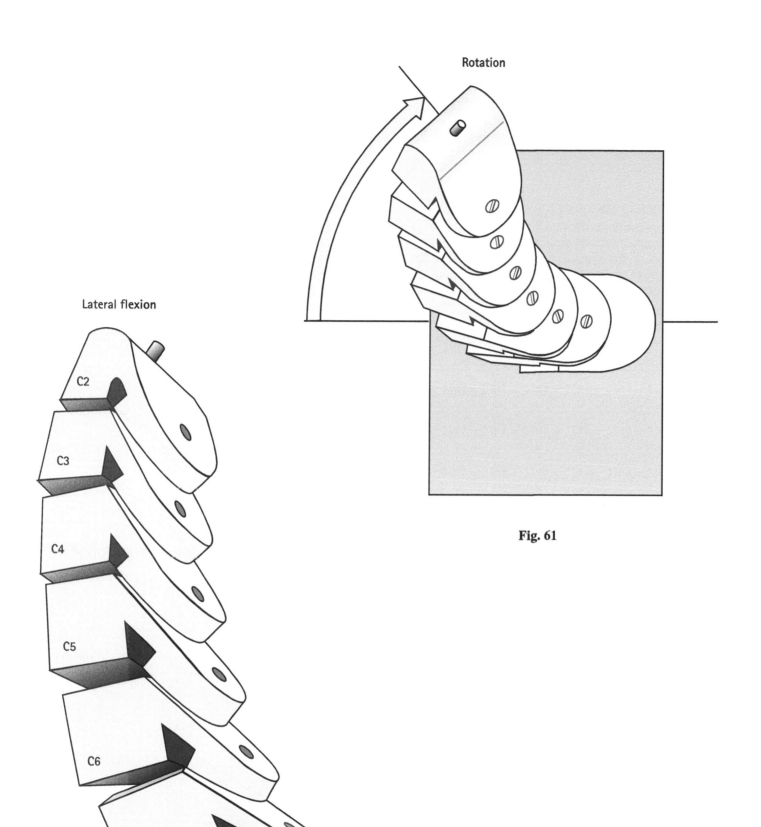

Rotation

Lateral flexion

C2
C3
C4
C5
C6
C7
T1

Fig. 60

Fig. 61

227

Comparison of the model and the cervical spine during movements of lateral flexion-rotation

An anterior view of the model (Fig. 62) reveals that the final phase of pure rotation produces a lateral flexion of 25° in the lower cervical spine during combined lateral flexion-rotation, i.e. its stereotypical movement. In **a radiograph taken strictly in the midsagittal plane** (Fig. 63), this lateral flexion can be seen to correspond exactly to a 25° lateral flexion of the axis with respect to the vertical plane.

From these two observations it can be concluded that, on the one hand, **movements of lateral flexion are always associated with rotation** in the cervical spine (as shown by Fick and Weber at the end of the nineteenth century) and, on the other hand (as more recently advanced by Penning and Brugger), that movements of lateral flexion in the lower cervical spine are *offset in the suboccipital* spine to produce pure rotation, and inversely that movements of rotation of the lower cervical spine are offset in the suboccipital spine to obtain pure lateral flexion (see Fig. 59, p. 225).

Fig. 63

25°

25°

C1
C2
C3
C4
C5
C6
C7

Fig. 62

Compensations in the suboccipital spine

A detailed diagram of the mechanical model of the cervical spine (Fig. 64) in the position of pure rotation illustrates the mechanical structure of the upper cervical spine and the compensating mechanisms destined to achieve pure rotation.

From top to bottom the following can be seen:
- the horizontal plate (A) representing the **basiocciput** (B)
- attached to the inferior surface of the basiocciput are two props in the coronal plane B, representing the **anteroposterior axis** (4) **of lateral flexion** of the atlanto-occipital joint articulating with the intermediate piece C. The **transverse axis** (3) **of flexion-extension** at the atlanto-occipital joint passes through this intermediate piece C, which is supported by the vertical strips D′ directly connected to the horizontal plate D. The latter rotates on plate E around a vertical axis (2), representing the axis of rotation of the atlanto-occipital joint (obscured by C in the diagram). Both axis 3 and 4 establish a **universal joint**.
- the plate E, which is *functionally equivalent to the atlas*, articulates with the axis vertebra F by a vertical piece 1 representing the dens and shown here as a partly tightened screw. This arrangement allows both movements of rotation and of flexion-extension on the convex superior surface of the axis F.

The diagram of the model (Fig. 64) also shows the mechanical elements corresponding anatomically to the various components of the suboccipital spine:
- the axis vertebra F with its dens corresponding to axis 1
- the atlas E articulating with the dens and the superior surface of the axis vertebra
- the occipital bone A, overlying a functional complex with three orthogonal axes corresponding to those of the atlanto-axial joint, i.e. the axis of rotation (2), the axis of flexion-extension (3) and the axis of lateral flexion (4). This is equivalent to a universal joint.

When the cervical spine is in a position of lateral flexion-rotation, pure rotation of the occipital bone is ensured by **three corrective movements**, which must take place in this suboccipital complex with its three axes and its three degrees of freedom:
- **rotation to the right around** axes 1 and 2 occurring mostly at the atlanto-axial joint (angle **a**) and at the atlanto-occipital joint (angle **b**)

- **extension** taking place around axis 3 (angle **c**) and offsetting the flexion that would occur as a result of pure rotation to the right on axis 1
- finally, a **small degree of lateral flexion in the opposite direction** (angle **d**) taking place around axis 4.

Anatomically speaking, the movements occur in the suboccipital spine with the help of the **small suboccipital muscles** (see p. 251), which can be called the **fine-tuners**, since they are strikingly similar to the **small control rockets** that maintain the orientation of a satellite relative to its fixed landmarks.

The complementary rotation of the suboccipital spine to the right is elicited (see p. 253) by the contraction of the obliquus capitis inferior, the right rectus capitis posterior major and the left obliquus capitis superior, which are also extensor muscles. Lateral flexion to the left is achieved by the left obliquus capitis superior, the left rectus capitis lateralis and the left rectus capitis anterior minor.

During **pure lateral flexion of the head** to the right (Fig. 59, p. 225) the component of counterrotation to the left is produced by contraction of the obliquus capitis inferior and the two left posterior recti; the **complementary lateral flexion** to the right is produced by the two right posterior recti and the right obliquus capitis superior. Finally, the **component of extension** produced by these three muscles is offset by the right longus capitis, rectus capitis anterior and rectus capitis lateralis.

Thus the mechanical model, which the reader can easily construct in a simplified version, makes it easier to understand the anatomical and functional link between the following:
- on the one hand, the lower cervical spine, which shows its stereotypical movement of torsion combining lateral flexion, rotation and extension and is equipped with muscles ideally situated for this type of movement, i.e. long muscles running an oblique course inferiorly, laterally and posteriorly
- on the other hand, the upper cervical spine, made up of an articular complex with three axes and three degrees of freedom and equipped with **fine-tuning muscles.**

Fig. 64

Ranges of movements of the cervical spine

By comparing **lateral photographs** taken in the extreme positions of **flexion-extension** (Fig. 65), it has been established that:
- the total range of flexion-extension in the lower cervical spine is 100-110° (LCS)
- the total range of flexion-extension for the entire cervical spine is 130° (ECS) with reference to the plane of the bite
- by subtraction, the range of flexion-extension in the suboccipital region is 20-30° (SOS).

Likewise, **anteroposterior views** taken in **lateral flexion** of the head (Fig. 66) show that the **total range of lateral flexion** is about 45°. By drawing a line joining the two transverse processes of the atlas and a line joining the bases of the mastoid processes, it can be deduced that the range of lateral flexion is about 8° in the suboccipital spine, i.e. **occurring solely in the atlanto-occipital joint.**

The **range of rotation** is more difficult to evaluate, especially as regards its various segmental components (Fig. 67). The total range of rotation on either side varies from 80° to 90°, including 12° in the atlanto-occipital joint and 12° in the atlanto-axial joint.

Fig. 65

Fig. 66

Fig. 67

Balancing the head on the cervical spine

The head is **perfectly balanced** when the **gaze is horizontal** (Fig. 68). In this position the plane of the bite (PB), shown here as a piece of cardboard held tightly between the teeth, is also horizontal, as is the auriculonasal plane (AN), which passes through the superior border of the external auditory meatus and the nasal spine.

Globally, the head corresponds to a **first-class lever:**
- the **fulcrum** (O) resides in the occipital condyles
- the **resistance** (G) is produced by the weight of the head acting through its centre of gravity near the sella turcica
- the **effort** (E) is provided by the posterior neck muscles as they must counterbalance the weight of the head, which tends to tilt forward as when a passenger falls asleep in a train.

The anterior location of the head's centre of gravity explains why the *posterior neck muscles are relatively more powerful* than the flexor muscles of the neck. In fact, the extensors counteract gravity, whereas the flexors are helped by gravity. This also explains why the posterior neck muscles are **always toni-cally active** to prevent the head from drooping forwards. When the body is lying down during sleep the tone of the muscles decreases and the head falls on the chest. The cervical spine is not straight but lies concave posteriorly, i.e. the **cervical lordosis**, which can be defined by the following:
- the **chord subtending the arc** (c) and corresponding to the straight line running from one occipital condyle to the ipsilateral postero-inferior corner of C7
- the **perpendicular** (p) joining the chord to the postero-inferior corner of C4.

This *perpendicular* increases with accentuation of the cervical curvature and equals zero when the cervical spine is straight. It can even become negative when during flexion the cervical spine becomes concave anteriorly. On the other hand, the *chord* is shorter than the full length of the cervical spine and equals it only when the cervical spine is straight. Thus a cervical index could be established along the lines of the Delmas index (see Chapter 1, p. 14).

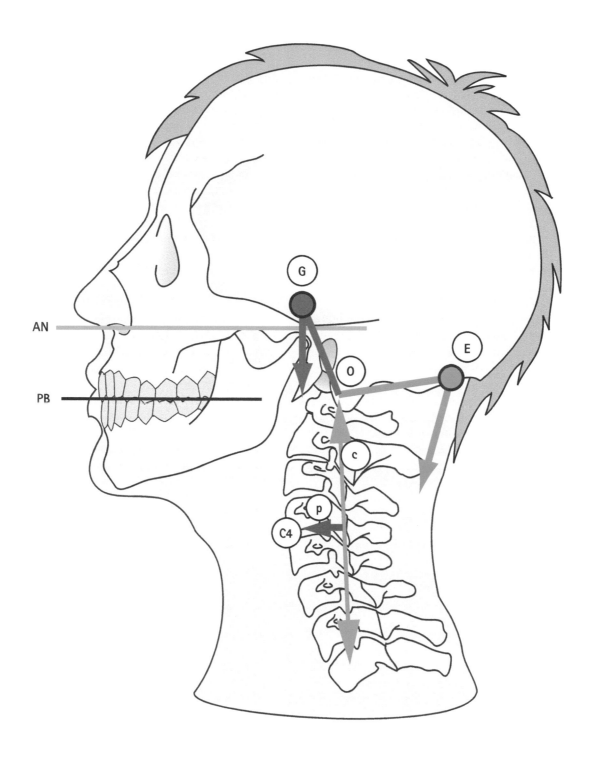

Fig. 68

Structure and function of the sternocleidomastoid muscle

This muscle should be called the sternocleido-occipitomastoid muscle, since it comprises four distinct heads (Fig. 69):

- a **deep head**, the **cleidomastoid** (Cm) stretching from the medial third of the clavicle to the mastoid process
- the other three heads can be teased out into an 'N' shape, but they are in reality very closely interwoven except in their inferomedial part near the medial end of the clavicle, i.e. **Sedilot's fossa**, where the cleidomastoid shows through.

These three superficial heads are:

- the **cleido-occipital** (Co), which overlies the bulk of the cleidomastoid and is inserted far back into the superior nuchal line of the occipital bone
- the **sterno-occipital** (So), which is closely associated with the sternomastoid and is inserted along with the cleido-occipital into the superior nuchal line
- the **sternomastoid** (Sm), which arises with the sterno-occipital by a common tendon from the superior margin of the manubrium sterni to be inserted into the superior and anterior borders of the **mastoid process.**

Globally, this muscle forms a wide and always clearly visible muscle sheet, stretched over the anterolateral surface of the neck and running an oblique course inferiorly and anteriorly. Its most conspicuous portion lies inferiorly and anteriorly and consists of the common tendon of the sterno-occipital and the sternomastoid.

The two sternocleidomastoid muscles form a fleshy fusiform mass clearly visible under the skin, and their two sternal tendons of origin border the suprasternal notch, which is always obvious regardless of the degree of portliness.

Unilateral contraction of the sternocleidomastoid (Fig. 70) gives rise to a complex movement with three components:

- contralateral **rotation** (R) of the head
- ipsilateral **lateral flexion** (LF)
- **extension** (E).

This movement raises the gaze and directs it to the side opposite to that of the contracting muscle. This position of the head is typical of **congenital torticollis**, which is often due to an abnormally *short* muscle on one side. We shall discuss in detail later (p. 265) the effects of concurrent bilateral contraction of the muscle, which vary according to the state of contraction of the other neck muscles as follows:

- *if the cervical spine is mobile*, this bilateral contraction **accentuates the cervical lordosis** with extension of the head and flexion of the cervical spine on the thoracic spine (see Fig. 99, p. 263)
- conversely, *if the cervical spine is kept rigid* and straight by contraction of the prevertebral muscles, then bilateral contraction produces **flexion of the cervical spine on the thoracic spine** and forward flexion of the head (see Fig. 100, p. 263 and Fig. 103, page 265).

Co

Sm

So

Cm

Fig. 69

LF

E

R

Fig. 70

237

The prevertebral muscles: the longus colli

The **longus colli** (Fig. 71) is the deepest of the prevertebral muscles and runs on the anterior surface of the cervical spine from the anterior arch of the atlas to C3. Anatomists mention **three parts:**

- an **oblique descending part** (d), attached to the anterior tubercle of the atlas and to the anterior tubercles of the transverse processes of C3-C6 by three or four tendinous slips
- an **oblique ascending part** (a), attached to the bodies of T2 and T3 and to the anterior tubercles of the transverse processes of C4-C7 by three or four tendinous slips

- the **longitudinal part** (l), lying deep to the former two parts and just lateral to the midline. It is attached to the bodies of T1-T3 and of C2-C7.

Thus the longus colli, on either side of the midline, carpets the whole anterior surface of the cervical spine. When both muscles contract simultaneously and symmetrically they *straighten the cervical curvature* and **flex the neck.** They are also critical in determining the static properties of the cervical spine.

Unilateral contraction produces **forward flexion** and **lateral flexion of the cervical spine on the same side.**

Fig. 71

The prevertebral muscles: the longus capitis, the rectus capitis anterior and the rectus capitis lateralis

These three muscles belong to the upper segment of the cervical spine (Fig. 72) and almost completely overlie the upper part (d, a and l) of the longus colli.

The longus capitis

As the most median of these three muscles, the longus capitis (lc) is in contact with its contralateral counterpart and is attached to the inferior surface of the basi-occiput in front of the foramen magnum. It overlies the upper part of the longus colli (d) and arises from the anterior tubercles of the transverse processes of C3-C6 by discrete tendinous slips.

It moves the suboccipital cervical spine and the upper part of the lower cervical spine. When both muscles contract together they **flex the head** on the cervical spine and **straighten the upper part of the cervical lordosis.** Unilateral contraction produces **forward flexion and lateral flexion of the head ipsilaterally.**

The rectus capitis anterior

The rectus capitis anterior (ra) lies posterior and lateral to the longus capitis and extends between the basi-occiput and the anterior surface of the lateral mass of the atlas up to the anterior tubercle of its transverse process. It runs obliquely, inferiorly and slightly laterally.

Its simultaneous bilateral contraction flexes the head on the upper part of the cervical spine, i.e. at the level of the **atlanto-occipital joint.** Its unilateral contraction produces a triple movement combining **flexion, rotation and lateral flexion** of the head ipsilaterally. These movements occur at the **atlanto-occipital joint.**

The rectus capitis lateralis

The rectus capitis lateralis (rl) is the highest of the intertransverse muscles and is attached above to the jugular process of the occipital bone and below to the anterior tubercle of the transverse process of the atlas. It lies lateral to the anterior rectus and overlies the anterior surface of the atlanto-occipital joint.

Its simultaneous bilateral contraction flexes the head on the cervical spine; its unilateral contraction produces a slight degree of lateral flexion ipsilaterally. Both these movements take place at the atlanto-occipital joint.

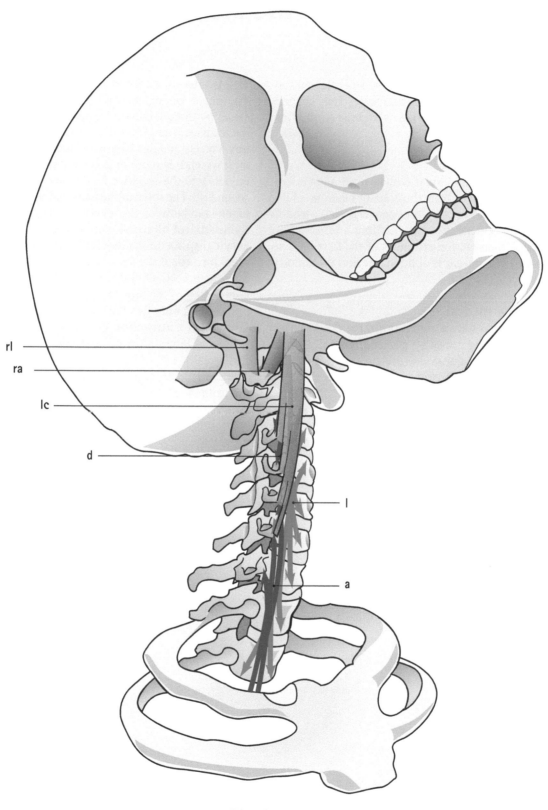

rl

ra

lc

d

l

a

Fig. 72

The prevertebral muscles: the scalene muscles

The three scalene muscles (Fig. 73) span the anterolateral surface of the cervical spine like true **muscular stays.** They connect the transverse processes of the cervical vertebrae to the first and second ribs.

The anterior scalene muscle

The anterior scalene (sa) is triangular with its apex lying inferiorly and arises by four tendons from the anterior tubercles of the transverse processes of C3-C6. Its fibres converge into a tendon for insertion into the scalene tubercle (Lisfranc's tubercle) on the upper surface of the anterior extremity of the first rib. The general direction of the muscle is oblique inferiorly, anteriorly and laterally.

The middle scalene muscle

The middle scalene (sm) lies in contact with the deep surface of the anterior scalene and arises by six tendinous slips from the anterior tubercles of the transverse processes of C2-C7, the lateral edges of the grooves in the transverse processes of C2-C7 and the transverse process of C7.

The muscle is flattened anteroposteriorly and is triangular with its apex located inferiorly. It runs obliquely, inferiorly and laterally to its insertion into the first rib just posterior to the **groove for the subclavian artery.**

The posterior scalene muscle

The posterior scalene (sp) lies posterior to the other two. It arises by three tendinous slips from the posterior tubercles of the transverse processes of C4-C6. Its fleshy belly is flattened transversely and lies lateral and posterior to the middle scalene, with which it is more or less continuous. It is inserted by a flat tendon into the superior border and the lateral surface of the second rib. The roots of the **brachial plexus** and the **subclavian artery** ran between the anterior and middle scalenes.

Symmetrical bilateral contraction of the scalenes **flexes the cervical spine** on the thoracic spine and **accentuates the cervical lordosis** if the neck is not kept rigid by the contraction of the longus colli. On the other hand, if the neck is held rigid by contraction of the longus colli, symmetrical contraction of the scalene **can only flex** the cervical spine on the thoracic spine.

Unilateral contraction of the scalenes (see Fig. 75, p. 245) produces lateral flexion and rotation of the cervical spine ipsilaterally.

The scalenes are also accessory inspiratory muscles when they act from their cervical vertebral attachments to elevate the first two ribs.

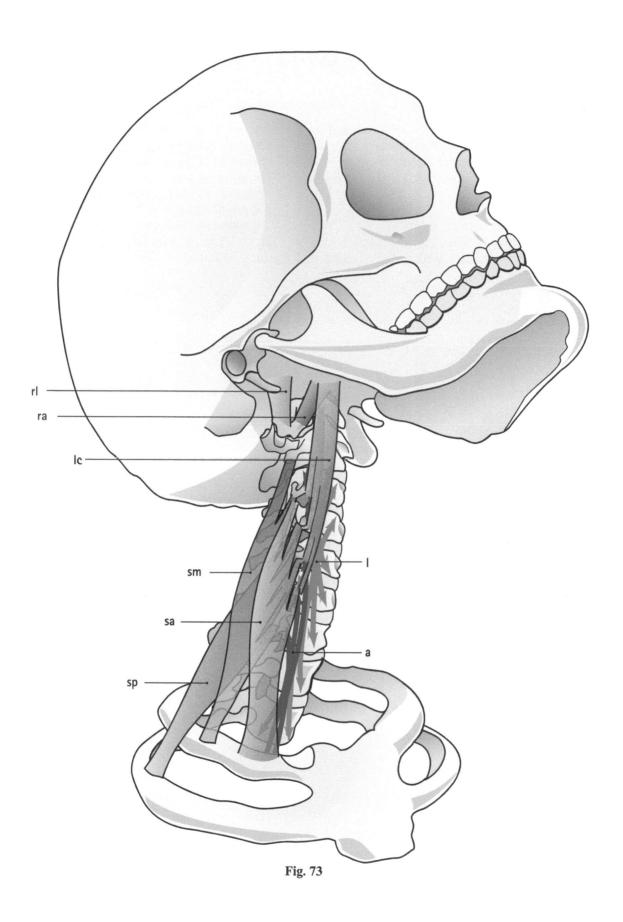

rl

ra

lc

sm

sa

l

a

sp

Fig. 73

Global view of the prevertebral muscles

On a frontal view of the cervical spine (Fig. 74, inspired by Testut) it is possible to localize all the prevertebral muscles:

- the **longus colli** with its longitudinal fibres (lcl), its oblique ascending (lca) and its oblique descending (lcd) fibres
- the **longus capitis** (lc)
- the **rectus capitis anterior** (ra)
- the **rectus capitis lateralis** (rl)
- the **intertransverse muscles** split into two planes – the anterior intertransverse muscles (ita) and the posterior intertransverse muscles (itp); their only action is to **flex the cervical spine ipsilaterally** (Fig. 75) with the help of the ipsilateral **scalene muscles**
- the **anterior scalene** (sa) is shown in toto on the right side with only its tendon included on the left in order to reveal the **middle scalene** (sm)
- the **posterior scalene** (sp) projects beyond the middle scalene only in its lower part near its insertion into the second rib.

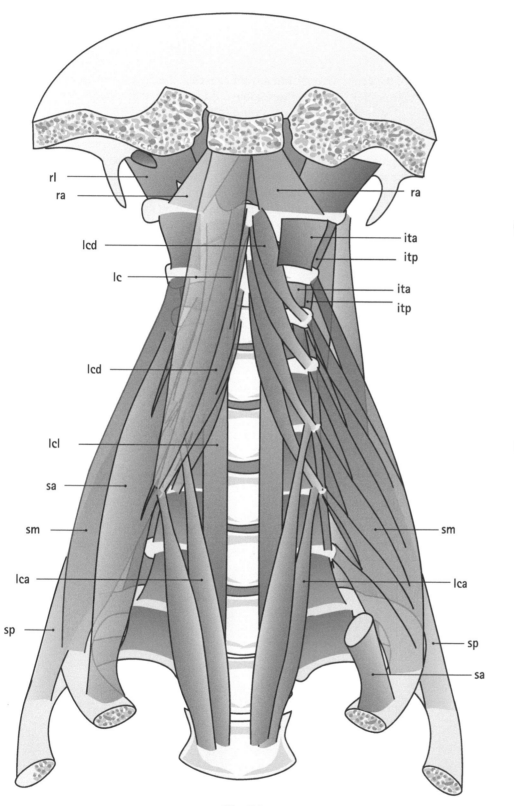

rl

ra

lcd

lc

lcd

lcl

sa

sm

lca

sp

ra

ita

itp

ita

itp

sm

lca

sp

sa

Fig. 74

Fig. 75

Flexion of the head and of the neck

Flexion of the head on the cervical spine and flexion of the cervical spine on the thoracic spine depend on the anterior muscles of the neck.

In the upper cervical region (Fig. 76) the rectus capitis anterior and the longus capitis **lca** produce flexion at the atlanto-occipital joint. The longus colli (lc 1 and lc 2) and longus capitis produce flexion in the lower vertebral joints. More important, the longus colli is vital for **straightening the cervical spine, holding it rigid** and correcting the lordosis (Fig. 77).

The **anterior neck muscles** (Fig. 78) are located at a distance from the cervical spine and thus work with a long lever arm; hence their strength as *flexors of the head and of the cervical spine*. These muscles are:

- the **suprahyoid muscles**: the **mylohyoid muscle** (mh) and the anterior belly of the **digastric muscle** (not shown here), which link the mandible to the hyoid bone

- the **infrahyoid muscles**: the thyrohyoid (not shown here), the sternocleidohyoid (sch), the sternohyoid (not shown here) and omohyoid (oh).

Simultaneous contraction of these muscles lowers the mandible but, when the mandible *is kept fixed by simultaneous contraction of the muscles of mastication*, i.e. the **masseter** (m) and the **temporalis** (t) muscles, contraction of the supra- and infrahyoid muscles produces flexion of the head on the cervical spine and flexion of the cervical spine on the thoracic spine. While simultaneously straightening the cervical curvature they exert a vital influence on the statics of the cervical spine.

Fig. 76

Fig. 77

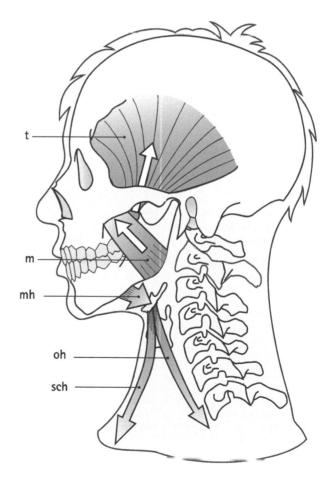

Fig. 78

The posterior neck muscles

Before studying the functions of the **posterior neck muscles** it is essential to have a full grasp of their distribution with the help of a **section taken in perspective** (Fig. 79), i.e. a **posterolateral view of the back of the neck from the right side** after resection of the superficial muscles in order to reveal the various planes.

The muscle planes

The back of the neck consists of **four muscle planes** superimposed on one another, which are as follows from deep to superficial:

- the deep plane with the suboccipital muscles and the muscles with multiple heads (see p. 256)
- the plane of the semispinalis capitis
- the plane of the splenius and levator scapulae
- the superficial plane.

The **deep plane** is directly adherent to the vertebrae and their joints and contains the small intrinsic muscles of the suboccipital cervical spine running from the occipital bone to the atlas and to the axis (also seen in Figs 80-82, p. 251):

- the **rectus capitis posterior major** (1)
- the **rectus capitis posterior minor** (2)
- the **obliquus capitis inferior** (3) and the **obliquus capitis superior** (4)
- the cervical portion of the **transversospinalis** (5)
- the **interspinales** (6) (see p. 256)

The **plane of the semispinalis** (partly resected) contains the following:

- the **semispinalis capitis** (7) (it is in part transparent and allows a view of 1-4)
- the **longissimus capitis** (8)
- more laterally, the longissimus cervicis, the longissimus thoracis and the **iliocostalis cervicis** (11).

The **plane of the splenius and of the levator scapulae** (also partly resected) contains the following:

- the **splenius** muscle divided into two parts, i.e. the **splenius capitis** (9) and the **splenius cervicis** (10). Only one of the three tendons of the cervicis (10′) is shown inserted into the posterior tubercle of the C3 transverse process. The other two tendons of insertion attached to the posterior tubercles of the transverse processes of C1 and C2 have been removed and are not shown here.
- the **levator scapulae** (12).

These muscles are tightly moulded onto those of the deep plane, around which they wrap themselves *as around a pulley*. Thus, when they contract they also produce a **significant degree of rotation of the head.**

The **superficial plane** comprises the following:

- mostly the **trapezius** (15) (almost entirely resected here)
- the **sternocleidomastoid**, which belongs to the back of the neck only in its posterosuperior part. It is shown partly resected to reveal its superficial (14) heads and its deep cleidomastoid head (14′).

In the depth of this plane the origins of the **middle and posterior scalenes** (13) can be seen through the gap between the muscles.

Global view

Except for the muscles of the deep plane, most of the posterior neck muscles are oblique inferiorly, medially and posteriorly and so produce at the same time **extension, rotation** and **lateral flexion** on the side of their contraction, i.e. exactly **the three components of the composite movement of the lower cervical spine** around the oblique axes previously described.

The **superficial plane**, on the other hand, comprises muscles that run in a counter direction to that of the intermediate muscles, i.e. obliquely, inferiorly, anteriorly and laterally. These muscles act not directly on the lower cervical spine but on the **head** and the **suboccipital cervical spine**, where, like the deeper muscles, they produce extension and lateral flexion ipsilaterally but *rotation contralaterally*. They are thus at once **agonists** and **antagonists** of the deep muscles, to which they are functionally complementary.

Fig. 79

The suboccipital muscles

The function of these muscles is underrated because they are not considered to be complementary to the muscles of the lower cervical spine. In real life these four **'Vernier'* muscles** are vital in establishing the position of the head by *reinforcing the wanted or eliminating the unwanted components* in the stereotypical triple movement of the lower cervical spine. A review of their anatomical arrangement makes it easier to visualize their direction in space and their functions. Three views of these muscles are needed:

- a **posterior view** (Fig. 80)
- a **left lateral view** (Fig. 81)
- a **posterolateral view in perspective from the right side and from below** (Fig. 82).

These figures show the following:

- The **rectus capitis posterior major** (1) is triangular in shape with its base located superiorly. It extends from the spinous process of the axis to the inferior nuchal line of the occipital bone. It runs an oblique course superiorly and slightly laterally and posteriorly.
- The **rectus capitis posterior minor** (2) is also triangular and flattened but shorter and deeper than the previous muscle and lateral to the midline. It extends from the posterior tubercle on the arch of the atlas to the medial third of the inferior nuchal line. Its oblique fibres run superiorly, slightly laterally and more directly posteriorly than the rectus capitis posterior major because the posterior arch of the atlas lies deeper than the spinous process of the axis.
- The **obliquus capitis inferior** (3) is an elongated, thick and fusiform muscle lying inferior and lateral to the rectus capitis posterior major. It extends from the lower border of the spinous process of the axis to the posterior margin of the transverse process of the atlas. Its oblique fibres run superiorly, laterally and anteriorly and thus cross in space the above-mentioned muscles, particularly the rectus capitis posterior minor (Fig. 82).
- The **obliquus capitis superior** (4) is a short, flat, triangular muscle lying behind the atlanto-occipital joint. It stretches from the transverse process of the atlas to the lateral third of the inferior nuchal line. Its oblique fibres run superiorly and posteriorly effectively in a sagittal plane, without any lateral orientation. It lies parallel to the rectus capitis minor and perpendicular to the inferior oblique (Fig. 81).
- The **interspinales** (5) lie on either side of the midline between the spinous processes of the cervical vertebrae **below the axis.** Thus they are equivalent to the two posterior rectus muscles.

---

* A 'Vernier' device, called after its inventor Pierre Vernier, can **increase considerably the accuracy** of any measuring instrument. Likewise, the small rockets used to *adjust precisely the orientation of a satellite* could be called 'Vernier' rockets. These 'Vernier' muscles could play a similar role in the **precise orientation of the head**.

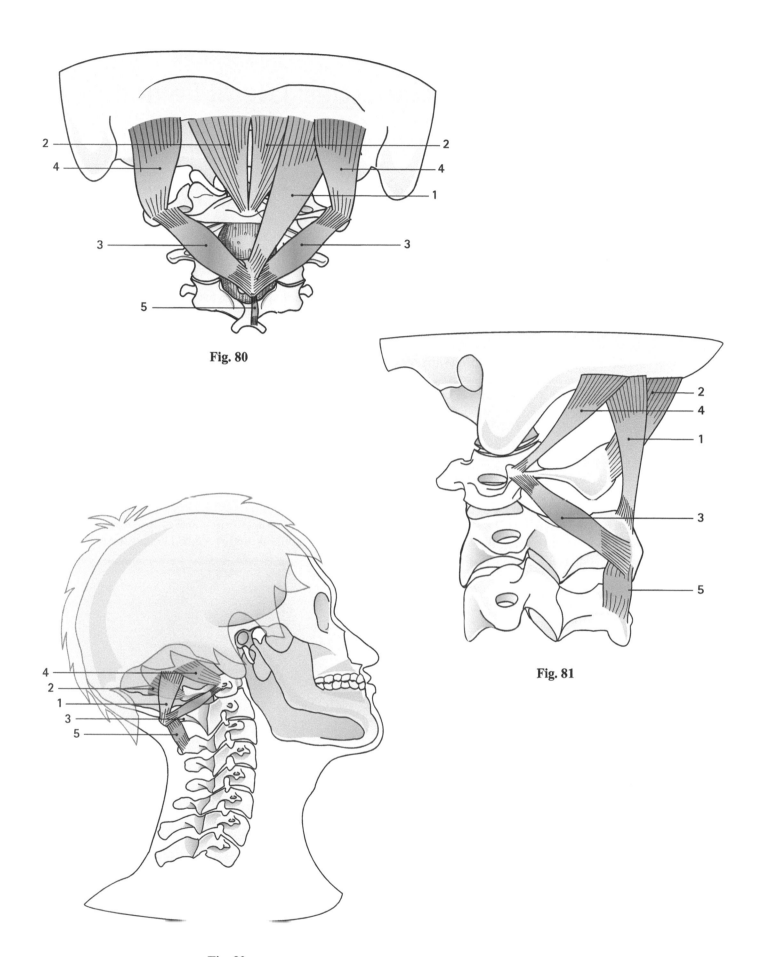

Fig. 80

Fig. 81

Fig. 82

Actions of the suboccipital muscles: lateral flexion and extension

By its location the **obliquus capitis inferior** plays an important role in the statics and dynamics of the atlanto-axial joint. A **left-side view** (Fig. 83) shows that the muscle *pulls back the transverse processes of the atlas*, and, as a result, its bilateral symmetrical contraction causes the atlas to recede into extension on the axis; this extension can be measured on oblique radiographs as the angle **a** at the level of the lateral masses of the atlas and angle **a'** at the level of its posterior arch.

A **superior view** (Fig. 84) clearly reveals this backward displacement **b**, produced by the symmetrical contraction of both inferior oblique muscles, which act like the arrow in a bow, inducing a forward displacement of the axis followed by a backward displacement of the atlas. This action reduces the tension in the transverse ligament, which passively checks the dens and prevents its posterior dislocation.

Rupture of the transverse ligament (Fig. 85) can only be of traumatic origin (black arrow), since normally the inferior obliques acting in concert play an important role in *maintaining the dynamic integrity of the median atlanto-axial joint.* Figure 86 (a superior view with superimposition of the vertebral canal of the atlas and the axis in lighter shade) illustrates the catastrophic consequences of such an instability in the atlanto-axial joint: the spinal cord is compressed, if not transected, as if by a cigar cutter or even a guillotine. The **grey-tinted area** represents the narrower canal with the compressed medulla oblongata inside. Unilateral contraction of the four posterior suboccipital muscles (Fig. 87, **posterior view**) produces lateral flexion of the head ipsilaterally at the atlanto-occipital joint. This angle of lateral flexion **f** can also be measured as the angle between the horizontal line passing through the transverse processes of the atlas and the oblique line joining the tips of the mastoid processes. The most efficient of these lateral flexors is undoubtedly the **obliquus capitis superior** (4), whose contraction elongates its contralateral counterpart by a distance **e.** It acts from the transverse process of the atlas, which is stabilized by the contraction of the **obliquus capitis inferior** (3). The **rectus capitis posterior major** (1) is less efficient than the superior oblique, while the efficiency of the **rectus capitis posterior minor** (2) is minimal as it lies too close to the midline.

Simultaneous bilateral contraction of the posterior suboccipital muscles (Fig. 88, **right lateral view**) extends the head on the upper cervical spine: this extension is produced at the atlanto-occipital joint by the rectus capitis posterior minor (2) and the obliquus capitis superior (4) and at the atlantoaxial joint by the rectus capitis posterior major (1) and the obliquus capitis inferior (3) (Fig. 87).

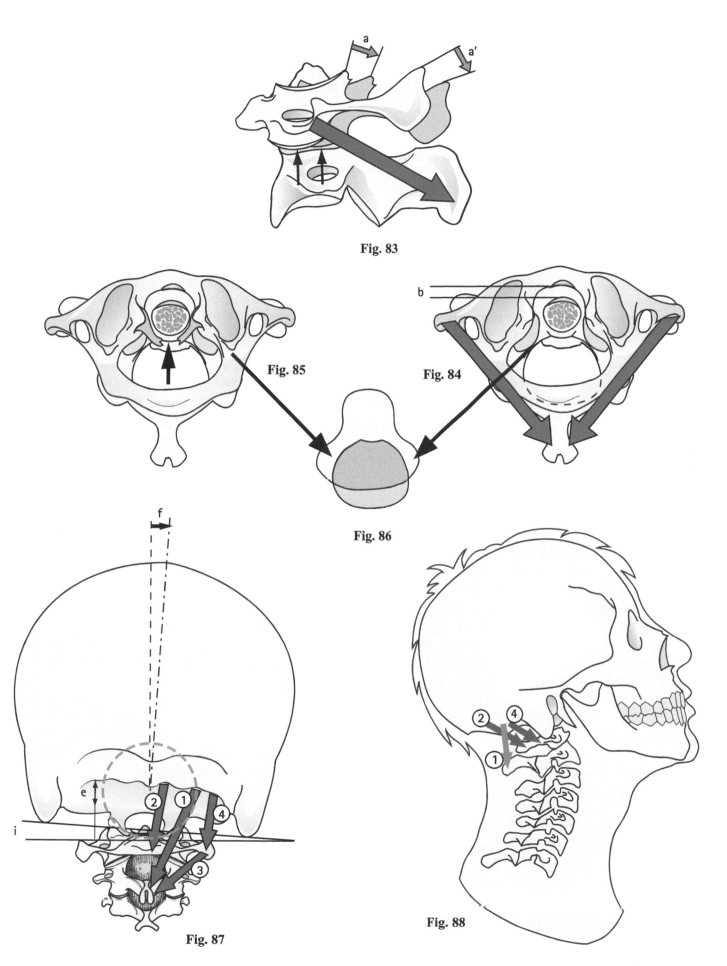

Fig. 83

Fig. 85

Fig. 84

Fig. 86

Fig. 87

Fig. 88

Rotatory action of the suboccipital muscles

In addition to extension and lateral flexion these muscles also produce rotation of the head.

Figure 89 (**inferior view of the upper level of the suboccipital region**, i.e. the atlanto-occipital joint) shows that contraction of the **obliquus capitis superior** (4) rotates the head 10° contra-laterally, i.e. contraction of the left superior oblique rotates the head to the right, as shown here. Consequently the right superior oblique (4′) and the right rectus capitis posterior minor (2) are passively stretched, and as a result they **restore the head to the neutral position.**

Figure 90 (**inferior view of the lower level of the suboccipital region**, i.e. the atlanto-axial joint with the outline of the atlas in red) shows that contraction of the rectus capitis posterior major (1) and the **obliquus capitis inferior** (3) rotate the head 12° ipsilaterally, i.e. contraction of the right rectus capitis posterior major (1) rotates the head to the right at both the atlanto-occipital and the atlanto-axial joints. Concurrently, the left rectus capitis posterior major is passively stretched over a distance of **a**

and, as a result, it helps restore the head to the neutral position. Contraction of the **right inferior oblique** (3) rotates the head to the right at the atlanto-axial joint.

Figure 91 (**a superior view in perspective taken from above and from the right side**) shows that contraction of the **oblique capitis inferior** (OCI), which runs diagonally between the spinous process of the axis and the right transverse process of the atlas, rotates the atlas to the left, while stretching the left rectus capitis major (Fig. 90) by a length **b**; this latter muscle then restores the head to the neutral position. The sagittal plane of symmetry **S** of the atlas also rotates 12° relative to the sagittal plane of the axis **A** when the obliquus capitis inferior contracts.

This detailed account of the actions of the suboccipital muscles makes it easier to understand how the unwanted components of lateral flexion or rotation are eliminated during pure movements of the head, as already demonstrated with the help of the mechanical model.

Fig. 89

Fig. 90

Fig. 91

The posterior neck muscles: the first and fourth planes

The deep plane of the posterior neck muscles

The deep plane contains the following:

- the **suboccipital muscles** (already described) in the upper cervical spine
- the **transversospinalis** or **multifidus* muscles** in the lower cervical spine.

These latter muscles are arranged symmetrically in the grooves formed by the spinous processes, the laminae and the transverse processes of the vertebrae from the atlas to the sacrum and consist of muscular slips overhanging one another like tiles on a roof.

There are two different accounts of the **arrangement of these muscular sheets** (Fig. 92):

- According to Trolard's traditional account (right side, T), the muscle fibres originate from the spinous processes and laminae of C2-C5 and converge onto the transverse process of C5.
- According to a more recent account by Winckler (left side, W) the muscle fibres run the other way from origin to insertion.

These two accounts are two different ways of describing the same anatomical fact, depending on whether the superior or inferior end is taken as the origin. Nonetheless, the fibres always ran an oblique course inferiorly, laterally and slightly anteriorly so that:

- **bilateral and symmetrical contraction** of the transversospinalis **extends** the cervical spine and **accentuates the cervical lordosis**; it is the erector muscle of the cervical spine
- **asymmetrical or unilateral contraction** produces extension, lateral flexion ipsilaterally and contralateral rotation of the cervical spine, i.e. movements similar to the head movements produced by the sternocleidomastoid. Thus *the transversospinalis is a synergist of the sternocleidomastoid*, but it acts segmentally along the cervical spine. On the other hand, the sternocleidomastoid with its similarly oriented fibres acts globally on the cervical spine, and its attachments at the two extremities of the spine constitute a **lever system with arms of considerable length.**

The superficial plane of the posterior neck muscles

The posterolateral **superficial plane** (Fig. 93) consists of the **trapezius** (2), which arises fanwise from a continuous line passing through the medial third of the superior nuchal line, the spinous processes of the cervical and thoracic vertebrae down to T10 and the posterior cervical ligament.

From this continuous linear origin the uppermost fibres run an oblique course inferiorly, laterally and anteriorly to be inserted into the lateral third of the clavicle, the acromion and the scapular spine. Thus the contour of the lower part of the neck corresponds to the **curved envelope** generated by the successive fibres of the trapezius. The trapezius plays an important role in the movements of the shoulder girdle (see Volume 1) but, when it contracts from the shoulder girdle as the fixed point, **it acts powerfully** on the cervical spine and the head as follows:

- **Symmetrical bilateral contraction** of both trapezius muscles **extends** the cervical spine and the head and **exaggerates the cervical curvature.** When this extension is thwarted by the antagonistic action of the anterior neck muscles, *they act as stays to stabilize the cervical spine.*
- **Unilateral or asymmetrical contraction** of the trapezius (Fig. 94, dorsal view, showing the **left trapezius** in contraction) produces **extension** of the head and of the cervical spine, **accentuation of the cervical curvature, lateral flexion** ipsilaterally and contralateral **rotation** of the head. The trapezius is therefore *a synergist of the ipsilateral sternocleidomastoid* (1).

The upper end of the sternocleidomastoid (1) is visible in the superomedial corner of the back of the neck (Fig. 93, **left side).** The external contour of the upper part of the back of the neck corresponds to the **curved envelope** formed by the successive fibres of the sternocleidomastoid (1) as they course inferiorly and twist around its axis.

---

* A multifidus muscle consists of multiple heads or lamellae.

Fig. 92

Fig. 93

Fig. 94

The posterior neck muscles: the second plane

The second plane, directly overlying the deepest plane (Fig. 95), comprises the semispinalis capitis, semispinalis cervicis, the longissimus thoracis, the longissimus cervicis and the upper part of the iliocostalis.

The **semispinalis capitis** (7), lying just lateral to the midline, forms a vertical muscular sheet interrupted by a tendinous intersection; hence the name 'digastric of the neck'. It arises from the transverse processes of T1-T4 and from the spinous processes of C7 and T1.

Its thick and rounded fleshy belly, overlying the transversospinalis, fills the vertebral groove and is separated from its contralateral counterpart by the ligamentum nuchae. Its convex lateral surface is closely applied to the two splenius muscles (9 and 10 in Fig. 96, p. 261). It is inserted into the squama of the occipital bone lateral to the external occipital crest (the inion) and between the two nuchal lines.

Bilateral symmetrical contraction of the semispinalis **extends** the head and the cervical column and **accentuates the cervical lordosis.**

Its unilateral or asymmetrical contraction produces **extension** combined with a slight degree of **lateral flexion** of the head ipsilaterally.

The longissimus capitis (8), lying lateral to the semispinalis capitis, is long and thin and runs obliquely, superiorly and slightly laterally. It arises from the transverse processes of C4-C7 and T1, and is inserted into the apex and posterior border of the mastoid process. Its fleshy belly is twisted on itself, since its lower fibres are inserted the most medially while its uppermost fibres, of cervical origin, are inserted the most laterally into the mastoid process.

Its bilateral symmetrical contraction extends the head; when this extension is checked by the antagonistic anterior neck muscles, the longissimus capitis stabilizes the head laterally just like an *inverted stay.*

Its unilateral or asymmetrical contraction causes **combined extension-lateral flexion** ipsilaterally (greater than that produced by the semispinalis capitis) and ipsilateral **rotation** of the head.

The long and thin longissimus cervicis (11), lying lateral to the longissimus capitis, arises from the apices of the transverse processes of T1-T5 and is inserted into the apices of the transverse processes of C3-C7. Its most medial fibres are the shortest, running from T5 to C7; its lateral fibres are the longest, running from T5 to C3.

Bilateral symmetrical contraction of both muscles extends the lower cervical spine; when this extension is prevented by their antagonists, they act as *stays.*

Unilateral or asymmetrical contraction produces **extension** of the head combined with **lateral flexion** on the same side.

The longissimus thoracis also belongs to the posterior neck muscles because its uppermost fibres are inserted into the transverse processes of the lowest cervical vertebrae. It is more or less continuous with the cervical part of the iliocostalis (11'), which arises from the upper borders of the upper six ribs and is inserted, along with the longissimus thoracis, into the posterior tubercles of the transverse processes of the five lowest cervical vertebrae. Its actions are similar to those of the longissimus cervicis; moreover, the cervical part of the iliocostalis acts as a *muscular stay* for the lower cervical spine and **elevates the upper six ribs** (see p. 162).

Fig. 95

The posterior neck muscles: the third plane

The **third plane** (Fig. 96) contains the splenius muscle and the levator scapulae lying deep to the trapezius.

The **splenius** (9 and 10), running from the skull to the thoracic region, arises from the spinous processes of C2-C7, the posterior cervical ligament, the spinous processes of T1-T4 and the interspinous ligament. Its fibres run an oblique course superiorly, laterally and anteriorly and wrap themselves around the muscles of the deep plane to be inserted as **two distinct bundles:**

• **the cephalic bundle or the splenius capitis** (9) is inserted below the sternocleidomastoid into the lateral half of the superior nuchal line of the occipital bone and into the mastoid process; it overlies incompletely the two semispinalis muscles, which can be seen through the triangle formed by the medial borders of the two splenius muscles

• **the cervical bundle or the splenius cervicis** (10) is shown on the left in relation to the splenius capitis and on the right side of the head by itself to illustrate how its fibres twist upwards to be inserted into the transverse processes of the atlas, axis and C3.

Symmetrical bilateral contraction of the splenius extends the head and the cervical spine and **accentuates the cervical curvature**.

Unilateral or asymmetrical contraction of the splenius produces combined ipsilateral **extension, lateral flexion** and **rotation**, i.e. the movement combination typical of the lower cervical column, as described on page 220.

The levator scapulae (12), lying lateral to the insertion of the splenius ceruicis, arises from the transverse processes of C1-C4. Its flattened belly wraps itself around that of the splenius but soon leaves it to run obliquely inferiorly and slightly laterally and gain insertion into the scapula.

When it acts from a fixed cervical spine it elevates the scapula; hence its name (see Volume 1), but when the scapula is kept fixed, it moves the cervical spine.

Bilateral and symmetrical contraction of both muscles extends the cervical spine and accentuates the cervical lordosis. When this extension is prevented, they act as stays to stabilize the cervical spine laterally.

Its unilateral or asymmetrical contraction, like that of the splenius, produces combined ipsilateral extension, unilateral rotation and lateral flexion, the movement combination typical of the lower cervical spine.

Fig. 96

Extension of the cervical spine by the posterior neck muscles

The posterior neck muscles are all **extensors of the cervical spine** but can be divided into **three groups** on the basis of their orientation.

Group I (Fig. 97)
This group comprises all the muscles attached to the transverse processes of the cervical vertebrae and running obliquely and posteriorly into the thoracic region:
- the splenius cervicis (1)
- the longissimus cervicis and the cervical portion of the iliocostalis (2)
- the levator scapulae (3).

These muscles extend the cervical spine and accentuate the cervical curvature. When they contract unilaterally they also produce ipsilateral extension, rotation and lateral flexion, i.e. the movement combination typical of the lower cervical column.

Group II (Fig. 98)
This group consists of all the muscles that run obliquely, inferiorly and anteriorly and thus in a direction opposite to those of group 1:
- on the one hand, the **transversospinalis muscular group** (4), which are intrinsic muscles of the lower cervical spine
- on the other hand, the muscles linking the occipital bone to the lower cervical spine: the **semispinalis** (6), the **longissimus capitis** (7) and the **splenius capitis** (not shown in the diagram)
- also the suboccipital muscles not included in the diagram (see pp. 250-254).

All these muscles extend the cervical spine, **accentuate the cervical lordosis** and **extend** the head on the cervical spine by virtue of their direct insertions into the occipital bone.

Group III
This group comprises all the muscles that bridge over the cervical spine without any attachments to the vertebrae and, as a result, unite the occipital bone and the mastoid process directly to the shoulder girdle. These muscles are the following:
- on the one hand, the **trapezius** (15 in Fig. 79, p. 249; 9 in Fig. 93, p. 257)
- on the other hand, the **sternocleidomastoid** (Fig. 99), which runs diagonally across the cervical spine. As a result, its bilateral and symmetrical contraction produces a combination of three movements: **extension** of the head on the cervical spine (10), **flexion** of the cervical spine on the thoracic spine (9) and **extension** of the cervical spine on itself with **accentuation of the cervical curvature** (11).

Thus the static properties of the cervical spine in the sagittal plane (Fig. 100) depend on a **constant dynamic equilibrium** between the following:
- on the one hand, **extension produced by the posterior neck muscles**, i.e. the splenius muscles (S), the longissimus cervicis, the iliocostalis, the longissimus thoracis (Lt) and the trapezius (T); all these muscles act like chords spanning the concavity of the cervical lordosis at various levels
- on the other hand, the **anterior and anterolateral muscles:**
  - the longus capitis (Lc), which flexes the cervical spine and straightens the cervical lordosis, and
  - the scalene muscles (Sc), which flex the cervical spine on the thoracic spine with a tendency to accentuate the cervical lordosis unless they are counteracted by the longus colli and the supra- and infrahyoid muscles (see Fig. 78, p. 247).

The simultaneous contraction of all these muscle groups **maintains the cervical spine rigid** in the intermediate position. Thus they act like *stays* located in the sagittal plane and in oblique planes. They are therefore essential in **balancing the head** and in supporting weights carried on the head, a common practice in certain populations for carrying loads while keeping the hands free. This practice undoubtedly strengthens the structural components of the cervical spine and increases the power of the neck muscles.

Fig. 97

Fig. 98

Fig. 99

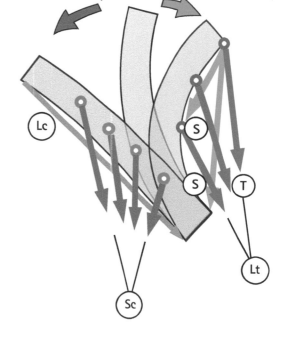

Fig. 100

Synergism-antagonism of the prevertebral muscles and the sternocleidomastoid muscle

Figure 99 (p. 263) illustrates perfectly the effects of symmetrical but isolated contraction of the sternocleidomastoid muscles (SCM). They cannot by themselves steady the head and the cervical spine. They need the assistance of synergistic-antagonistic muscles that set the stage by first straightening the cervical curvature (Fig. 101). These muscles are the following:

- the **longus colli** (Lc), lying just anterior to the vertebral bodies, straightens the cervical lordosis *because it is located on its convexity*
- the **suboccipital muscles**, which flex the head on the cervical spine (Fig. 102): the **longus capitis**, the **rectus capitis anterior** and the **rectus capitis lateralis**
- finally, the **supra- and infrahyoid muscles**, which lie anterior to the cervical spine and act at a distance with the help of a long lever arm, provided the mandible is pressed against the maxilla by contraction of the muscles of mastication.

Once the **cervical spine is kept rigid**, the **cervical lordosis straightened** (Fig. 103) and extension of the head on the cervical spine is prevented by the anterior suboccipital muscles and the supra- and infrahyoid muscles, **simultaneous contraction** of the two sternocleidomastoids (Fig. 104) produces **flexion** of the cervical spine on the thoracic spine. Thus there are multiple instances of synergism-antagonism between the sternocleidomastoids and the prevertebral muscles lying immediately anterior to the spine or at a distance from it.

When loads are carried on the head all these muscles are contracted simultaneously to achieve the constant dynamic equilibrium that transforms the head and neck into a single structure, both rigid and flexible, as it lies on top of the spine. This is the triumph of bipedalism!

We strongly recommend this exercise to women who desire to acquire the gait of a queen.

Fig. 101

Fig. 103

Fig. 102

Fig. 104

The ranges of movements of the cervical spine taken as a whole

There are many ways of measuring the ranges of these global movements. For flexion-extension and lateral flexion they can be measured with precision on lateral and frontal radiographs, but it is more difficult to measure the range of rotations without the use of the CT scan or the MRI.

Surface markings, however, can also be used, and for **flexion-extension** (Fig. 105) the reference plane is the plane of the bite, which is horizontal in the neutral position. It can be established by biting on a sheet of cardboard, which then represents the plane of the bite. The range of extension (E) is then given by an angle which is open superiorly and is formed by the plane of the bite and the horizontal plane. The range of flexion (F) is given by an angle which is open inferiorly and is formed by the plane of the bite and the horizontal plane. These ranges have already been defined but are very variable from one subject to another.

Rotation of the head and neck (Fig. 106) can be measured when the subject sits in a chair with the shoulder girdle kept in a strictly steady position. The reference plane is then taken as the intershoulder line, and rotation is measured as either the angle **R** between the reference plane and the coronal plane passing through the ears or by the angle **R'** between the midsagittal plane of the head and the midsagittal plane of the body. With the subject lying supine on a hard surface, more precise measurements can be made with the use of the **angle gauge*** placed on the forehead in the transverse plane.

Lateral flexion (LF) is measured by the angle formed by the interclavicular line and the interocular line (Fig. 107).

Flexion-extension and lateral flexion can be measured more precisely with the use of an **angle gauge** placed on the head in the sagittal plane for flexion-extension or in the coronal plane for lateral flexion.

There is also another head movement rarely used in the West but common among **Balinese dancers** (Fig. 108), i.e. lateral translation of the head (T) without any lateral flexion. Some women can perform this movement as a social accomplishment; it is considered successful only *if the interocular line stays parallel to itself.* To understand this movement it is essential to have a thorough grasp of the mechanics of the compensatory movements at the suboccipital joints, which were discussed at the start of this chapter. The clue to this movement is the ability to perform counter-counter-compensations. Thus, start with the lower cervical spine positioned in right lateral flexion-rotation-extension, and then perform at the suboccipital articular complex a counter-rotation to the left, a slight flexion and, above all, a counter-inclination to the left to restore the nasal meridian to the vertical plane. The competition is open!

NB: It is very easy to perform this movement of the Balinese dancers on the mechanical model of the cervical spine (see p. 319).

---

* The angle gauge is sparingly used in articular physiology, and yet it measures the angle formed with the vertical plane, a potentially useful feature. On the other hand, it is included in the instrument panel of commercial planes, where it monitors the lateral inclination of the plane.

Fig. 105

Fig. 106

Fig. 107

Fig. 108

Relationship of the neuraxis to the cervical spine

The central nervous system lies inside the cranium and the vertebral canal. The cervical spine protects the lower medulla oblongata as it emerges through the foramen magnum and the spinal cord, which gives off the nerve roots for the cervical and brachial plexuses.

Thus the medulla and the cervical cord are closely related to the highly mobile parts of the cervical spine, especially in the suboccipital region, which is a very special **zone of mechanical transition** (Fig. 109, **viewed in perspective from the front and the right side**). In fact, as the medulla (M) exits through the foramen magnum to become the spinal cord (SC), it lies between and slightly behind the occipital condyles (C and C′), which provide the **two supports for the head** as it rests on the cervical spine. Between the occipital condyles and C3, however, the atlas and the axis will redistribute onto three columns the weight of the head, initially supported by the two condylar columns (C and C′). These three columns, which span the entire spine, are the following:

- **the main column**, formed by the vertebral bodies (1) in front of the spinal cord (hidden in the diagram, as it lies behind [2])
- **the two minor lateral columns** formed by the articular processes (2 and 3) lying on either side of the cord.

The lines of force are split at the level of the axis, which is a veritable **distributor of forces** between the head and the atlas on the one hand and the rest of the cervical spine on the other. **A right lateral view** (Fig. 110) shows that the loads supported by each of the occipital condyles (C) will split into two components:

- anteromedially, the more important **static component** directed towards the vertebral bodies (VB) via the body of the axis
- posterolaterally, the **dynamic component** directed towards the column of the articular processes (A) via the pedicle of the axis and the inferior articular process lying below the posterior arch of the axis.

This suboccipital region therefore is at once the **pivot**, i.e. the *most mobile area of the spine* and the area of *maximal mechanical activity*. This stresses the significance of the ligaments and bony structures involved in stabilizing this region. The most critical bony structure is the **dens**. A fracture at its base makes the atlas totally unstable on the axis, which can then tilt backwards or *forwards* with more serious consequences, e.g. anterior dislocation of the atlas on the axis with compression of the medulla and sudden death.

Another important structure for the stability of the atlas on the axis is the **transverse ligament**. Rupture of this ligament allows anterior dislocation of the atlas on the axis, while the intact dens moves backwards to compress and severely damage the medulla (see Figs 84-86, p. 253). Ruptures of the transverse ligament occur more rarely than fractures of the dens.

In the lower cervical spine the zone of maximal activity lies between C5 and C6, where anterior dislocations of C5 and C6 occur most frequently with the **inferior articular facets of C5 becoming hooked** onto the superior facets of C6 (Fig. 111). In this position the cord is crushed between the posterior arch of C1 and the posterosuperior angle of the body of C6. Thus, depending on the level of the cord lesion, paraplegia or a potentially rapidly fatal quadriplegia may result.

It goes without saying that all these lesions, which render the spine very unstable, can be *made worse by injudicious handling*, especially *when injured persons are picked up*.

Thus any flexion of the cervical spine and of the head on the cervical spine can aggravate compression of the medulla or of the cord. Therefore, when an injured person is picked up, one of the rescuers must be solely responsible for *the gentle and continuous traction of the head along the axis of the spine* and carry it *slightly extended* so as to prevent the displacement of any possible fracture in the suboccipital region or below.

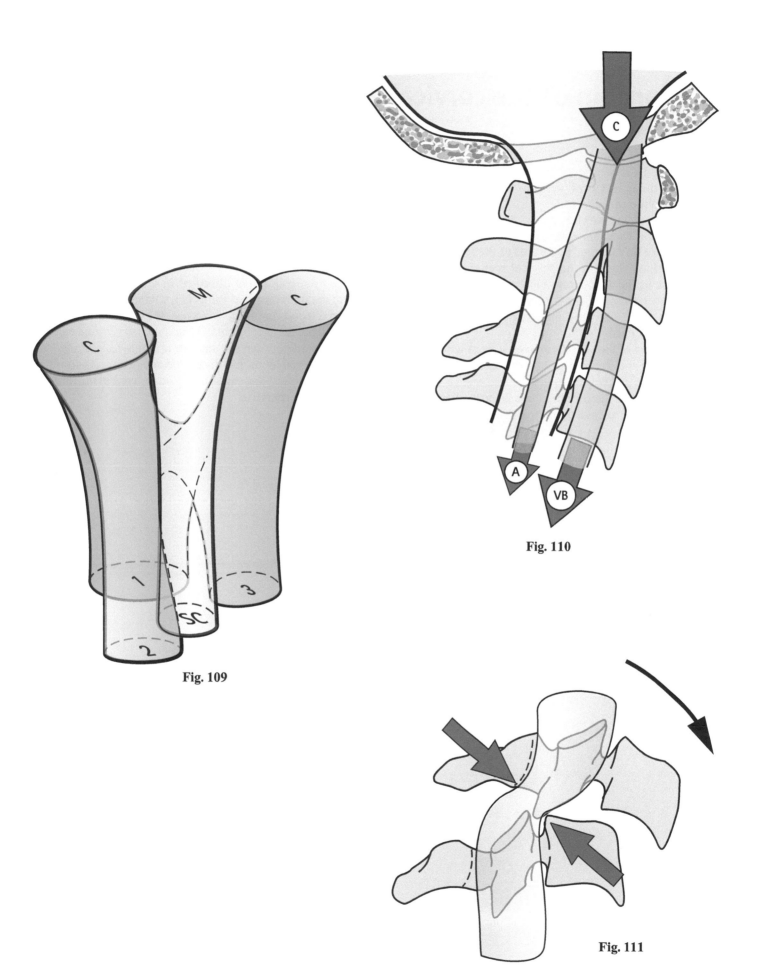

Fig. 109

Fig. 110

Fig. 111

Relationship of the cervical nerve roots to the spine

Having studied the relationship of the cervical spine to the medulla and the spinal cord, we now turn our attention to its relationship to the nerve roots.

At every level of the cervical spine, the cervical nerve roots emerge from the canal through the **intervertebral foramina.** These roots can be damaged by **lesions of the spine** (Fig. 112). **Disc herniation** is rare in the cervical region as the postero-lateral escape of the disc (arrow 1) is impeded by the presence of the uncinate processes. Thus, when they occur, they are more central (arrow 2) than in the lumbar region and so tend to **compress the spinal cord.**

Note the location of the **vertebral artery** (red) with its venous plexus (blue) in the foramen transversarium of the transverse process.

Cord compression in the cervical spine is more often caused by osteoarthritis of the uncovertebral joints (arrow 3).

Figure 113 (**left lateral view of the cervical spine**) shows the close relationship between the cervical roots exiting through the intervertebral foramina and the **facet joints** posteriorly and the **uncovertebral joints** anteriorly (upper part of diagram). During the early onset of cervical osteoarthritis (lower part of the diagram), osteophytic excrescences grow not only on the anterior borders of the vertebral discal surfaces (1), but also more prominently (as observed in three-quarter radiographs) from the uncovertebral joints (2), whence they project into the intervertebral foramina. Likewise, the osteophytes grow posteriorly from the facet joints (3), and the nerve roots can become compressed between the anterior osteophytes coming from the uncovertebral joints and the posterior osteophytes coming from the facet joints. This explains the **nerve root symptoms of cervical osteoarthritis.**

Fig. 112

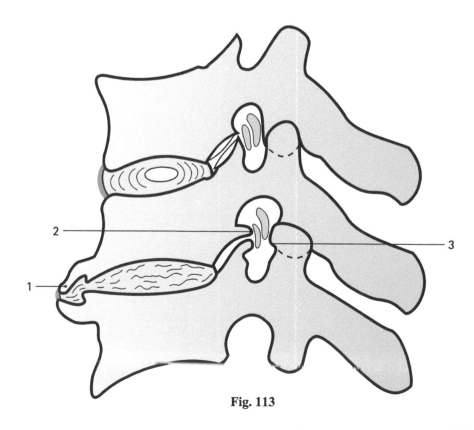

Fig. 113

The vertebral artery and the neck blood vessels

We think it is important to define precisely the *close relationship of the vertebral artery to the spine* and to outline in general terms its relationship to the neck vessels, which *supply the brain and the face*.

The **head and neck blood vessels** arise from the aortic arch (Fig. 114, right lateral view):

- on the **right side** they arise directly from the brachiocephalic trunk (1), which then divides into the right subclavian artery (2) and the right common carotid artery (3)
- on the **left side** they arise separately from the left common carotid artery and the left subclavian artery.

The vertebral artery (4′) arises from the subclavian artery and traverses the supraclavicular groove on its way to the foramen transversarium of C6. It then ascends (4) in a canal formed by the **successive vertebral foramina transversaria** until it reaches the atlas (Fig. 115, seen from behind and the right). Just above the **transverse process of the atlas** (Fig. 116) it changes direction completely and forms an arch (6) which skirts the back of the lateral mass of the atlas, where it lies in a deep groove. Thus it enters the vertebral canal (4) in close contact with the lateral surface of the brainstem and of the medulla and runs superiorly, anteriorly and medially to join its contralateral counterpart to form the important **basilar artery** (5), which lies on the anterior surface of the brainstem as it passes through the foramen magnum and enters the posterior fossa.

All along its course the *vertebral artery is exposed to injury*:

- first, *in the canal formed by the foramina transversaria* it must slide freely to be able to accommodate the changes in the curvature and direction of the spine (it can be damaged by displacement of any vertebra relative to its neighbours)
- then, *on its way to join its mate*, it is in contact with the dens, from which it is separated by the transverse ligament.

It is worth noting that the formation of the basilar artery, which will itself divide into two, illustrates Occam's principle of parsimony* since both vertebral arteries could easily have gone through the foramen magnum.

Moreover (Fig. 114), the common carotid artery (3) ascends on the anterolateral aspect of the neck and divides into the following:

- the external carotid artery (9), which then divides into the superficial temporal artery (10) and the maxillary (11) to supply the face
- the internal carotid artery (7), which ascends to the base of the skull and into the cranial cavity, where it forms a U-bend (8) before dividing into its terminal cerebral branches.

The important point to bear in mind is that the basilar artery anastomoses with the internal carotid arteries at the **circle of Willis.** Thus vertebral arteries **supply not only the structures in** the **posterior fossa**, i.e. the cerebellum and the brainstem, but also the **anterior cerebrum** in cases of carotid arterial insufficiency.

Hence this essential role of the vertebral arteries underscores the importance of safeguarding them during any manipulations on the cervical spine. *The vertebral artery is known to have been injured during somewhat vigorous manipulations of the cervical spine.*

---

* William of Occam was a famous monk, a scholastic theologian, an English philosopher and logician, also known as 'the invincible doctor'. He was bom at Ockham, Surrey, *c.* 1290, was excommunicated in 1330 and died of the plague in Munich in 1349. He introduced the principle of parsimony or universal economy, i.e. 'The truth of a theory must be based on the least number of preconditions, reasons and demonstrations'. This principle is also known as 'Occam's razor', since it cuts out all unnecessary preconditions from the demonstration during a logical discussion. Copernicus as a thinker is a descendant of Occam, in that he showed that the Ptolemaic system was too complicated to explain the retrograde movement of the inner planets, and thus solved the problem by introducing the heliocentric system. Like Einstein he was sensitive to the beauty of demonstrative reasoning.

Fig. 115

Fig. 116

Fig. 114

The importance of the vertebral pedicle: its role in the physiology and pathology of the spine

At all spinal levels the **vertebral pedicle** plays an essential mechanical role in **unifying the vertebral bodies**, which support the spine at rest, and the **vertebral arch**, which protects the neuraxis and is critical during movements since it gives attachment to the muscles.

The pedicle is a **tubular structure** consisting of a strong cortex and a medullary cavity filled with cancellous bone. This relatively short cylinder is variably orientated in space depending on the level of the spine but shares some constant features.

It is clearly visible in an **oblique radiograph** (Fig. 117) as the eye of the 'Scottie dog' (cross) but on careful scrutiny it can also be seen **along the full length of the spine** (Fig. 118). Thus each vertebra 'has two eyes' and one must learn to 'look the vertebrae in the eye'. Hence the extremely ingenious idea of Roy-Camille (1970) of inserting a screw into the axis of the pedicle in order to unify the posterior arch and the vertebral body or to provide a **zone of solid support** in one or more vertebrae (Fig. 119). Preoperative radiographs will reveal any possible deviations of the pedicle and allow the horizontal insertion of a screw from the back in the **sagittal plane** (Fig. 120).

This technique is not recommended to novices in spinal surgery. Landmarks must first be established precisely for the selection of the point of insertion, and then the direction of insertion must also be defined according to the spinal level. This direction is horizontal **in the lumbar region** (Fig. 121) but may sometimes be slightly oblique medially. Until now the skill and experience of the surgeon ensured the right orientation of the screw, taking into account the proximity of the nerve roots exiting via the intervertebral foramina above and below (Fig. 122). Nowadays the **use of computers** makes the approach more precise and allows the screw to be inserted with greater safety. Perhaps computer technology will allow the insertion of these screws elsewhere in the spine, especially in the cervical region (Figs 123-125), where the pedicles are much thinner and run in different directions. At present screws can be inserted only at the level of C2 and C7.

The introduction of the pedicule screw constitutes a **very important step in spinal surgery**, e.g. in the stabilization of fractures, in the placement of plates and of zones of support for one or more vertebrae. This **innovative idea** is the result of a **perfect knowledge of anatomy.**

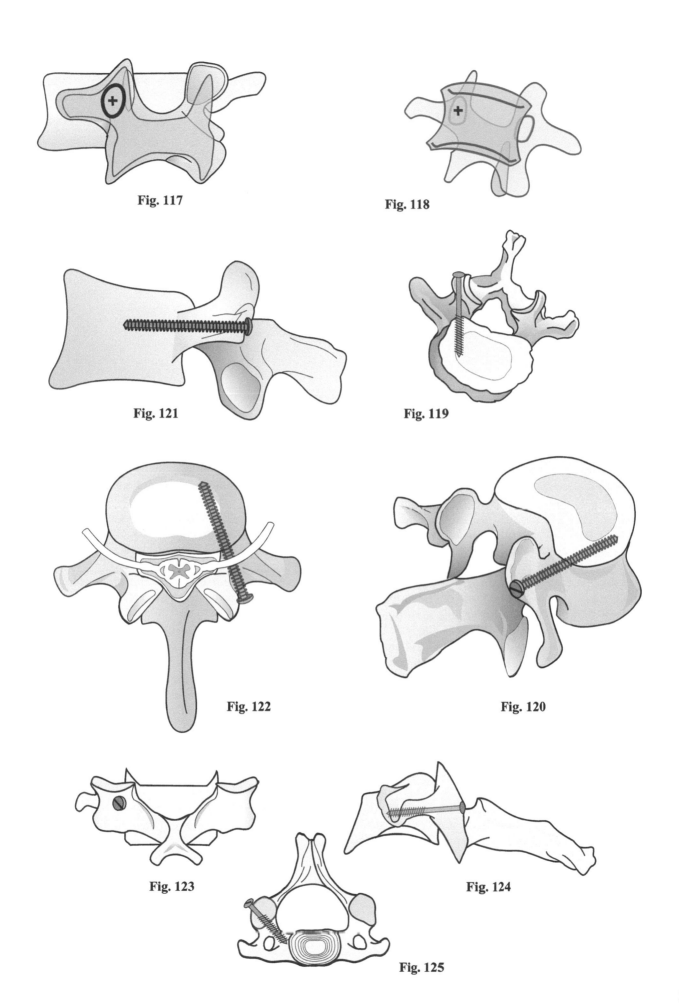

Fig. 117

Fig. 118

Fig. 121

Fig. 119

Fig. 122

Fig. 120

Fig. 123

Fig. 124

Fig. 125

Chapter 6

THE HEAD

The head crowns the **spine** and contains our most precious organ – the brain – our **central computer**, which is protected inside the solid bony **cranium.** The cranium is attached to the spine, which contains the **spinal cord**, a bundle of nerve fibres transmitting information to and from the entire body. It is ovoid and consists of lamellar bones articulating among themselves at **immobile bony sutures.**

The **face**, which is part of the skull, contains **two major sensory organs**, i.e. the eyes and the ears, which are responsible for information about the environment. The closeness of these sensors *shortens the time needed for transfer of data to the brain*; this is yet another example of Occam's razor. The mobility of the **cervical spine** allows these **sensory organs to be properly oriented in space** and thus increases their efficiency.

The head contains **two portals of entry** for food and air:

- The **mouth** is rightly placed *below the nose*, which can thus monitor the **smell of food** before it is ingested. Food is also monitored by the **taste buds**, which determine its *chemical nature* and through intuition or the collective memory of the species reject the ingestion of noxious or toxic substances.
- The **nose** *controls, filters and warms up the inspired air.* The upper airway *crosses the digestive tract* at the level of the pharynx and of the larynx. The larynx possesses a **protective valve** with an extremely precise mechanism that prevents the introduction of solid or liquid material into the airways. The human **larynx** (see p. 184 for a description of its physiology) plays a vital role in **phonation**, i.e. in modulating sounds,

which are then articulated by the mouth and the tongue. Thus humans enjoy a communication system using sound, i.e. **language**, which allows the sharing of information and feelings. This oral transfer is supplemented by the use of the *written* word. The head also contains **muscles and joints** of an unusual type. The superficial muscles of the face (studied in detail by Duchenne de Boulogne) do not act on any skeletal structures. They are the muscles of facial expression and provide a **quasi-international second mode of communication** supplementing the oral mode. These **orbicular** muscles control facial orifices: the *orbicularis oris* closes the mouth and the *orbicularis oculi* closes the eyes. On the other hand, there is only a *dilator naris*.

The external acoustic meatus stays open and is helped in the gathering of sounds by the *auricle*, which cannot be oriented in space as in animals.

There are also bones for the transfer of vibrations between the eardrum and the internal ear, i.e. the **auditory ossicles of the internal ear** (not discussed any further here). Furthermore, there are **two synovial joints**, i.e. the **temporomandibular joints**, allowing the movements of the mandible, which are essential for feeding and phonation. Finally, there are *two boneless joints*, which involve the intraorbitar eyeballs and control the orientation of the gaze.

In the following pages (see p. 296) we shall deal with the temporomandibular joints and the mobility of the eyeballs (see p. 306).

The cranium

The cranial skeleton (Fig. 1) comprises *22 flat bones*, which are derived from the osseous anlagen in the 12 cranial somites but have been profoundly altered to fit their specific functions, i.e. formation of the cranium and of the face.

The **cranium** is made up of bony plates, which consist of an intermediate layer of *spongy bone* (the diploe) sandwiched between two very strong layers of compact bone, i.e. the *epicranial table* externally and the *endocranial table* internally. At the base of the skull these flat bones blend with more massive bones, which connect it to the face and the cervical spine.

The **ovoid cranium** is made up of six bony plates:

- The **occipital bone** (1) lies posteriorly and has a wide squama forming the occiput. It is continuous with the basilar process (the basiocciput), which is perforated by *the foramen magnum* for the passage of the medulla and the spinal cord into the vertebral canal. On each side of the foramen magnum lie its *two condyles*, which articulate with the cervical spine at the level of the atlas.
- The **parietal bones** (2) are two symmetrical bony plates forming the superolateral part of the cranium and articulating posteriorly with the occipital bone.
- The **frontal bone** (3) is an unpaired, shelllike plate across the midline forming the forehead and articulating posteriorly with the parietal bones. Anteriorly it contains the *supraorbital margins* continuous posteriorly with the *upper walls of the orbits*.

These four bones constitute the *cranial vault*.

The **basicranium** is made up anteroposteriorly of the following:

- The **ethmoid bone** (4) is an unpaired midline bone, which lies behind the central part of the frontal bone and makes up the bulk of the *nasal fossae*. Its upper part contains the **cribriform plate** perforated by olfactory sensory nerves before they join the two **olfactory bulbs**. The body of the ethmoid contains many air sinuses which make it lighter, and in the sagittal plane lies its vertical plate separating the *two nasal fossae* which harbour the *superior and middle conchae*.
- The **sphenoid bone** (5) is an unpaired midline bone, and its body unites the ethmoid and the occipital. It is the most complex bone of the basicranium and can be compared to a *biplane* with the fuselage corresponding to the body of the sphenoid. In the upper part of the body is located the *pilot's seat*,* corresponding to the **sella turcica.** The **two lesser wings** above articulate with the frontal bone and the **two greater wings** below form the floor of the temporal fossa. These two sets of wings are separated by the superior orbital fissures located at the back of the orbit. The bilateral **pterygoid processes** correspond to the landing gear of the biplane.
- The **temporal bone** (6) borders the cranium bilaterally with its *squama*, and the basicranium with its *pyramidal petrous part*.
- Each **palatine bone** (7) articulates with the pterygoid process of the sphenoid and forms part of the *nasal fossa* and of the *palate*.
- Each **zygomatic bone** (8) contributes to the wall of the orbit and corresponds to the *cheekbone*.
- The **two nasal bones** (9) meet in the midline to form the *nasal bridge*.
- Each **maxilla** (10) forms by itself the bulk of the **facial skeleton** on one side. It encloses the *maxillary sinus* and so is almost hollow. It forms the *floor of the orbit* and its lower part contains the **superior alveolar process** and the *palatine process*, which makes up most of the palate.
- The **mandible** (11) is a midline, unpaired, horseshoe-shaped bone with two *ascending rami* supporting the **condyles** or **condylar processes**, which contain the mobile articular surfaces of the **temporomandibular joint.** It contains the **inferior alveolar process**, which is the counterpart of the superior alveolar process.

For the sake of completeness the small bones, i.e. the **vomer**, the **lacrimal bone** and the **inferior concha** deserve mention, but they play no structural role in the cranium and are not shown here.

Detailed description of these bones and their relations can be found in textbooks of descriptive anatomy.

---

* The pilot corresponds to the pituitary gland, which is the conductor of the endocrine orchestra.

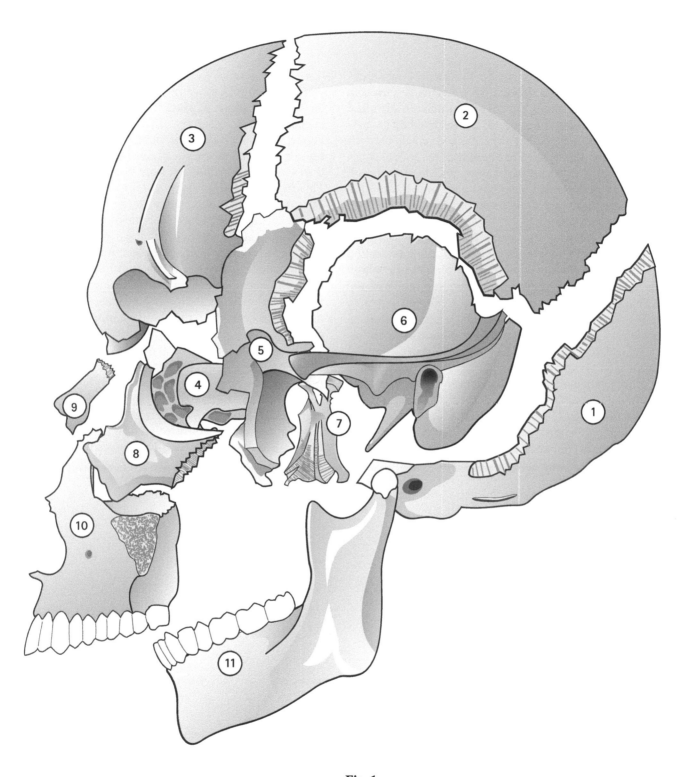

Fig. 1

Drawings based on Andràs Szunyoghi's work.

The cranial sutures

Except for the maxilla and the mandible the cranial bones articulate among themselves by **sutures.** In the fetus and even in the neonate the cranial bones are not united and are therefore **relatively mobile among themselves**, as illustrated by the persistence of the anterior fontanelle, which is completely ossified only at 8-18 months after birth. The mobility of the cranial bones in the young child is the result of the *rapid growth of the brain*, which continues postnatally. Subsequent bone growth can keep pace with that of the brain until adolescence, when the skull reaches its full development.

The **bony sutures**, which join together the bony plates (Fig. 2), are extremely *wavy*, so that, when they are tightly **interlocked** (Fig. 3), no movement can take place in the **plane of the plate.** A comparison with a **puzzle** (Fig. 4) illustrates very well the snug fit among the pieces (Fig. 5), provided that they stay in the *same plane*, i.e. resting on the table. On this basis traditional anatomy teaches that these sutures are **completely immobile.** Nowadays this dogma is challenged by certain specialists, who try to explain a whole host of diseases in terms of sutural motion. On a closer look it becomes obvious that movements among the pieces of the puzzle can only occur *outside the plane* (Fig. 6). The cross-section (Fig. 7) shows clearly that any sliding movement is possible only at right angles to the plane.

As shown in Figure 1 on page 279, most of these sutures are **not perpendicular to the plane** but are **variably oblique.** *It is therefore impossible for the plates to slide obliquely one on the other* (Fig. 8) in a movement of subduction, in keeping with the **theory of tectonic plates** proposed by Wegener (Fig. 9) to explain earthquakes.

Figure 1 does not rule out the possibility that the obliquity of the sutures would allow the squamous portions of the two temporal bones to *glide laterally* as it were in a movement of expansion. This theory of *cranial bone tectonics* remains to be proved in experiments involving anteroposterior compression of the head (without using the torture technique of the Inquisition!) and the use of coronal densitometric CT scans before and after compression. Then there will still be the problem of explaining the physiopathology that could result from sutural mobility. The research could be done on anatomical specimens. Plain logic favours the notion of micromovements in these sutures since, if they were absent, these *sutures would have disappeared during evolution.*

The skulls of hominids, in particular among the primates and Homo sapiens, contain a feature characteristic of the *transition to the erect posture.* In animals, e.g. the **dog** (Fig. 10, the skull outlined in blue and the face in red), four-footedness ensures that the cervical spine is nearly horizontal and the foramen magnum lies inferocaudally. Conversely, during evolution, **bipedalism** (Fig. 11) led to an **antero-inferior shift of the foramen magnum** in Homo sapiens, i.e. *to a position below the cranium.*

Fig. 4

Fig. 5

Fig. 6

Fig. 2

Fig. 3

Fig. 7

Fig. 8

Fig. 9

Fig. 10

Fig. 11

The cranium and the face

The skull (Figs 12 and 13) comprises within a single structure the **cranium** (blue line) containing the **brain**, our **central computer** (where reside our personality and our individuality), and the **face** (red line), containing the main **sensory organs** (i.e. for sight, taste, smell and hearing), which provide information about the environment. The proximity of these sensors to the brain, which handles the data, *shortens the time of information transfer.* It is another example of the principle of parsimony (Occam's razor), which states that maximal efficiency is achieved with the use of a minimum of parts.

The mobility of the head, provided by the **cervical spine**, allows the **sensory organs to be oriented in space** and improves their efficiency, as does their **elevated position** secondary to **bipedalism.** Inside the cranium the **cerebellum** is an essential link in the coordination and the fine-tuning of messages coming from the cerebrum. The cerebrum *makes the decisions* and the cerebellum *allows them to be carried out.*

The head also contains **two portals of entry** (Fig. 14): the mouth for food and the nose for air.

The **mouth** is rightly placed **below the nose**, which can first monitor the **smell of food** before it is ingested. Food is then monitored by the **taste buds**, which determine its chemical nature through intuition or collective memory of the species or knowledge of their poisonous contents can reject noxious or toxic substances. **Mastication** carried out by the **mandible** allows the mouth to **crush and grind** food and mix it with saliva to make it more digestible.

The **nose** *controls, filters and warms up inspired air*; its role in filtration is essential. Because of the placement of the portals of entry and the *anterior location of the lungs* and the *posterior location of the digestive tract*, the **upper airways cross the upper digestive tract at the levels of the pharynx and of the larynx.** The larynx provides an extremely precise mechanism of closure for the **glottis** and the **epiglottis** and acts as a **protective valve** that prevents the introduction of even the smallest amount of solid or liquid material into the airways. In humans the **larynx** (see p. 182 for an account of its physiology) also plays a vital role in **phonation** by modulating sounds that are then articulated by the mouth and the tongue. Thus human beings enjoy a communication system using sound, i.e. **articulate language**, which allows the sharing of information, knowledge, experiences, commands and feelings.

The head is therefore a remarkable and wonderful example of functional integration. It also contains **joints** (i.e. the temporomandibular joints) and **muscles** of an unusual type. These muscles of **facial expression** provide a **second quasi-international system of communication** supplementing the oral form and transmitting mainly feelings and emotions. It can betray what is expressed by mouth.

Fig. 12

Fig. 13

Fig. 14

The visual field and localization of sounds

The head lies on top of the spine, and **its rotation has a range of close to 180°**, thus greatly improving the efficiency of vision and hearing. This rotation allows the head with its sensors to move in the direction of the source of the stimulus *without having to move the body*, which is not the case with animals without necks, like fish.

The visual field
In the neutral position (Fig. 15, A) the **visual field** has a range of close to 160° (a). The visual fields of the eyes overlap in front of the head and provide a **sector of stereoscopic vision** for the hands to work. If the head turns (H) to the right (r) or to the left (l), the entire visual field (T) is significantly increased to 270°, with only a **blind sector of 90°** (P) posteriorly. Some animals with very long necks like the giraffe can survey the entire field of 360° simply by rotating their necks.

Sound localization
The **localization of the source of a sound** (Figs 16 and 17) is the result of the lateral placement of the ears, which are *separated by the cranium*. A sound source lying **outside the plane of symmetry** (Fig. 16) is not perceived in the same way by both ears:

- The ear on the side opposite to the source (S) perceives a sound *slightly attenuated* by the presence of the face, which is an obstacle to be bypassed.
- This same ear therefore perceives a sound *out of phase* with that perceived by the other ear. The path taken by the sound is slightly longer; hence the *phase difference* (d).

When the head is instinctively turned towards the side where the sound is louder (Fig. 17), the *intensity of the sound becomes the same and the phase difference disappears*. At this point the sound source (S) lies exactly in the plane of symmetry of the head, and the eyes can **telemetrically** (see p. 310) measure the distance to the source, if it can be identified at all. It is interesting that this process of sound localization **works as well at the back as in front of the head** though less efficiently, a tremendous advantage for the localization of an unexpected threat!

Fig. 15

Fig. 16

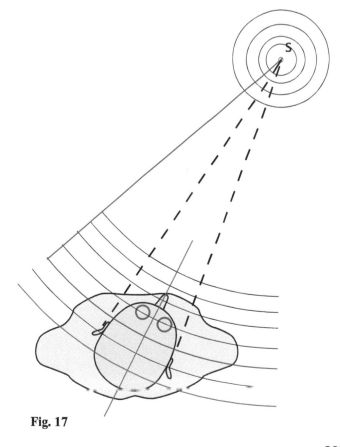

Fig. 17

The facial muscles

The facial muscles are very special and different from the other muscles of the locomotor system, which interlink bones; *the facial muscles do not move any bones*. They are inserted into one of the cranial bones only on one side, and even then *some of them have no direct attachments to the bones*. In fact, they are inserted into the deep surface of the dermis and move the skin. Their function has received special attention from Duchenne de Boulogne. Their first and **main function** is to **control the facial orifices** by closing or opening them, particularly the eyes and the mouth, and to a lesser degree the nose; the external acoustic meatus is not involved at all.

Their **second function** is to **change facial expression** in order to externalize and **express feelings**. They do so in accordance with a **universal language**, which is understood all over the world and supplements or sometimes contradicts the spoken word. This facial language is almost always accompanied by a **universal set of expressive gestures**, mostly with the hands. These muscles can be described in detail *around the orifices they control*, i.e. the eyes, the nose and the mouth (Figs 18 and 19).

Around the eyes

The **orbicularis oculi** has an *orbital part* (2) and a *palpebral part* (3). Contraction of this *sphincteric muscle* closes the eyelids. Thus, closing the eyes is an active process: even during sleep the orbicularis maintains enough tonic activity to keep the eyes closed. This tonic activity is lost with death: one needs to close the eyes of a dead person. In everyday life, the rapid and automatic and unconscious closure of the eyelids, i.e. **blinking**, is very important in **keeping the eyeballs moist** with tears.

- Opening the eyes is also an active process carried out by the **levator palpebrae superioris**, which lies within the orbit (see Fig. 32, p. 307).
- Between the eyes and at the root of the nose there are two muscles, the **procerus** (4) and the **corrugator supercilii** (5),

which allow one to frown and bring the eyebrows closer together.
- Above the eyebrows lies the **frontalis** (1), which moves the scalp *forwards*. It forms a digastric muscle with the **occipitalis** (1') by sharing a common tendon inserted into the *epicranial aponeurosis,* which supports the scalp. The occipitalis moves the scalp *backwards*.

Around the nostrils

In addition to small **dilator muscles** (not shown here) there are the **nasalis** (6), which wrinkles the nose, and the **levator labii superioris alaeque naris** (7).

Around the mouth

The **orbicularis oris** (12) is also a sphincter with no bony attachments. It closes the mouth.

All the other muscles open the mouth as follows:

- by elevating the upper lip like the **levator anguli oris** (8), which contracts to reveal the canine tooth
- by pulling it upwards and outwards, i.e. the **zygomaticus minor** (9) and the **zygomaticus major** (10)
- by pulling the labial commissures outwards, i.e. the **buccinator** (17) and the **risorius** (13), which is inserted into the **masseter** (11), one of the muscles of mastication like the **temporalis** (18). They attenuate the lips, allowing them to *vibrate* in the mouthpiece of the trumpet, which was called buccina in post-classical Latin; hence the word **buccinator** (*trumpeter* in Latin) for the muscle
- by depressing the corner of the mouth, i.e. the **depressor anguli oris** (14), which is the muscle used to show contempt
- by depressing the lower lip, i.e. the **depressor labii inferioris** (13) involved in kissing
- as for the **mentalis** (16), it puckers the skin over the chin, the first stage of sorrow before the tears.

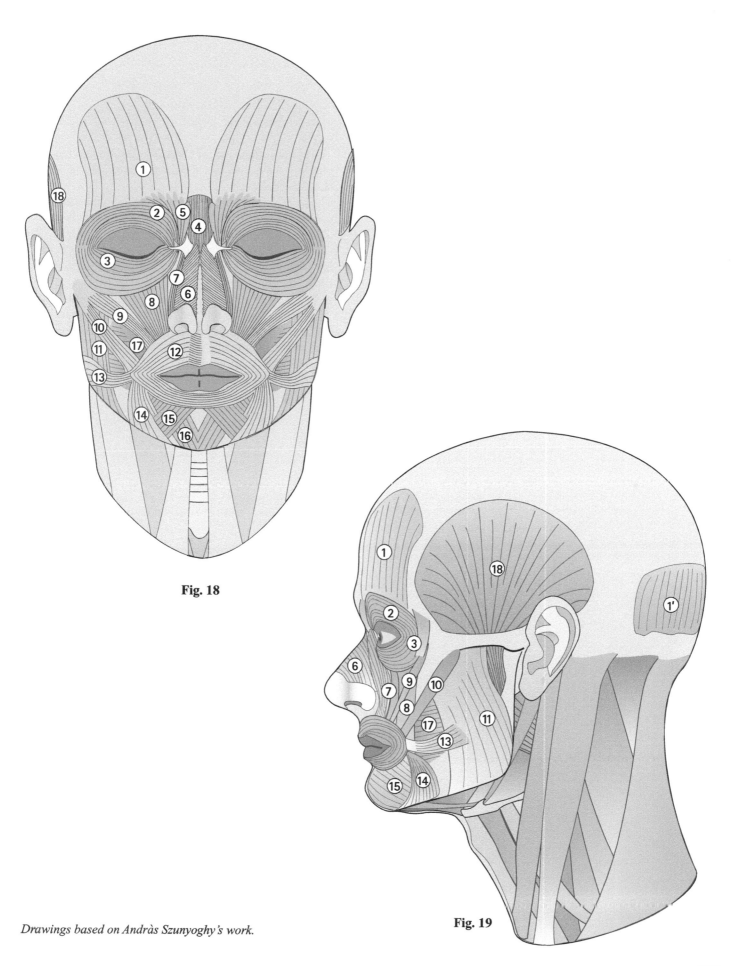

Fig. 18

Fig. 19

Drawings based on Andràs Szunyoghy's work.

The movements of the lips

Lips are crucial in all stages of **feeding**, i.e. opening the mouth, taking hold of the food with the lips and then closing the mouth during chewing. When one gets ready to drink, the lips move forward towards the glass. No animals, except monkeys, can perform this gesture, and this is why the higher mammals drink with the tongue by lapping up the liquid.

The mouth plays an important part in **facial expression**, e.g. in joy, contentment, contempt, hatred, disgust, doubt and refusal. All these feelings and many more are first expressed by the shape of the mouth.

The mouth also takes part in certain expressions of emotion, as in a **kiss** or during **singing.**

Rounding the mouth allows the emission of sounds like **whistling.** The inability to whistle is a **test for facial paralysis.** These movements are controlled by the following muscles:

- The **zygomaticus major** (Fig. 20) elevates and pulls supero-laterally the corners of the mouth, producing a **smile with the mouth closed.**
- The **buccinator** (Fig. 21), lying deep, and the **risorius**, lying superficial, are very strong in pulling outwards the corners of the mouth, thus **thinning down the lips** and allowing them to *vibrate* during blowing. This is how one plays any instrument with a mouthpiece, like the trumpet, the horn or the trombone.

A smile (Fig. 22) is the result of opening the mouth halfway, as the **zygomatic muscles** and the **risorius** pull its corners upwards and outwards and the **depressor labii inferioris** and the **mentalis** depress the lower lip.

Finally (Fig. 23), contraction of the **depressor anguli oris** pulls down the corners of the mouth to express **contempt.**

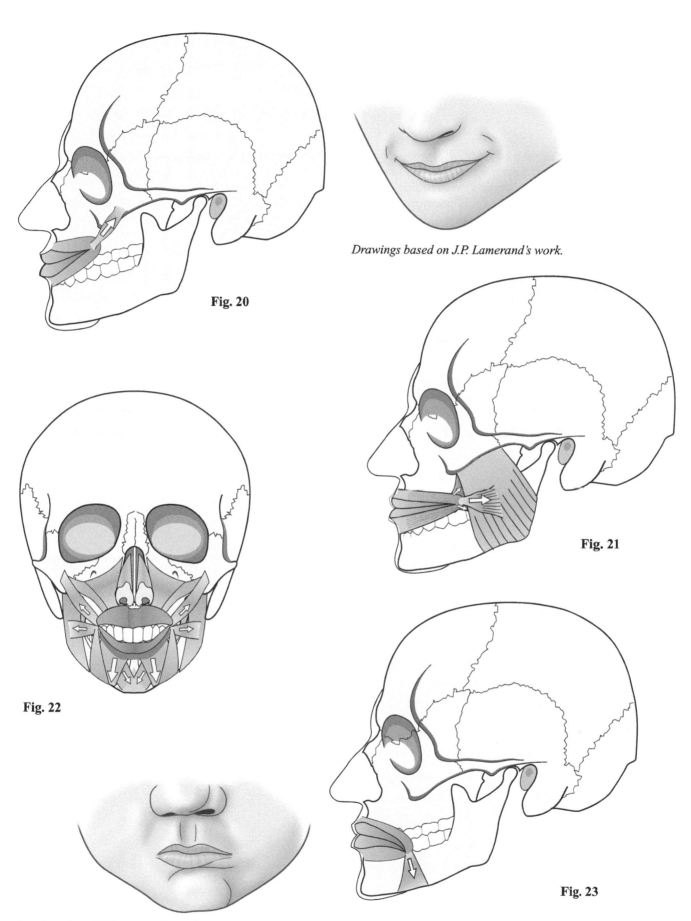

Fig. 20

Drawings based on J.P. Lamerand's work.

Fig. 21

Fig. 22

Fig. 23

Drawings based on J.P. Lamerand's work.

Lip movements (continued)

When the mouth is half open as for a **smile** (Fig. 24), opening it wide or almost closing it allows the pronunciation of the vowels **A** and **I** respectively. Saying 'cheese' at the time of being photographed ensures that the mouth is in the smile position.

On the other hand, a greater degree of contraction of the **orbicularis oris** (Fig. 25) rounds up and closes the mouth to allow **E** or **O** or even **U** to be voiced.

In the position for pronouncing the French **U** the mouth is maximally closed and rounded, and the muscles that close and widen it are then fully contracted.

In Figure 25 the left eye is shut by contraction of the palpebral part of the orbicularis oculi, and one can imagine that the subject is winking while whistling.

Fig. 24

A

Drawings based on J.P. Lamerand's work.

I

E

O

U

Drawings based on J.P. Lamerand's work.

Fig. 25

Facial expressions

Here are a few facial expressions chosen from the commonest; they will allow readers to test their recently acquired knowledge of the subject. For each expression readers can train themselves to describe the various movements involved. The answers are included upside down in each section.

Disgust (Fig. 26)

- Around the mouth
  – lowering of the corners of the mouth by contraction of the depressor anguli oris
  – puckering of the chin by contraction of the mentalis.
- Around the eyes
  – partial closure of the eyes by contraction of the orbicularis oculi
  – frowning by contraction of the corrugator supercilii.

Weeping (Fig. 27)

- Around the mouth
  – lowering of the corners of the mouth by contraction of the depressor anguli oris
  – slight contraction of the orbicularis oris
  – puckering of the chin by contraction of the mentalis, but to a lesser degree than during the expression of disgust.
- Around the eyes
  – no contraction of the orbicularis oculi
  – frowning by contraction of the corrugator supercilii.

Fatigue (Fig. 28)

- Around the mouth
  – lowering of the corners of the mouth by contraction of the depressor anguli oris
  – puckering of the chin by the mentalis but to a lesser degree than during the expression of disgust
  – relaxation of the palpebral part of the orbicularis oris.
- Around the eyes
  – no contraction of the orbicularis oculi
  – raising of the eyebrows by contraction of the frontalis.

The smile (Fig. 29)

- Around the mouth
  – elevation of the corners of the mouth by the zygomaticus major, the zygomaticus minor and the risorius
  – curling of the lower lip by contraction of the depressor labii inferioris
  – relaxation of the orbicularis oris.
- Around the eyes
  – contraction of the orbital and palpebral parts of the orbicularis oculi
  – elevation of both alae nasi by the contraction of the levatores labii superioris alaeque nasi.

Anger (Fig. 30)

- Around the mouth
  – curling of the upper and lower lips by contraction of the levator anguli oris and of the depressor anguli oris, respectively
  – elevation of each nostril by contraction of the levator labii superioris alaeque nasi.
- On the nose
  – contraction of the nasalis, procerus and corrugator supercilii.
- Around the eyes
  – contraction of the orbital part of the orbicularis oculi
  – elevation of the upper eyelid by contraction of the levator palpebrae superioris
  – elevation of the eyebrows by contraction of the frontalis.

Fig. 26

Fig. 27

Fig. 28

Fig. 29

Fig. 30

Drawings based on J.P. Lamerand's work.

293

The temporomandibular joints

The temporomandibular joints receive little attention, but they are of **vital importance**, since *without them eating is impossible.* They allow movements of the mandible, which articulates with the base of the cranium (Fig. 31) by **two ellipsoid joints** (black arrow) sited just in front of and below the external acoustic meatus **A**. These **mechanically linked** joints cannot function one without the other and are essential for **mastication.**

The body of the **mandible** (1) is shaped like a transversely flattened *horseshoe*, and its superior border (2) bears the **inferior alveolar process** (3). Its posterior border is continuous with **two ascending rami** (4), which terminate each in a **condyle** (5) supported by a **narrow neck** (6). Anterior to the condyle, the ramus terminates in the transversely flattened **coronoid process** (7).

Movements of the mandible are **complex** and are shown diagrammatically by six arrows:

- The simplest movement takes place **vertically** and includes:
  - **jaw opening** (O), which allows food to be introduced between the two alveolar ridges
  - **jaw closing** (C), which allows the food to be held and *chewed.*
- **A side-to-side** movement (S) to the right or to the left, which allows the surfaces of the inferior and superior molars to slide on one another like a **millstone** for the purpose of *crunching and crushing food.*
- **A longitudinal anteroposterior movement**, i.e. **protrusion** (P) and **retraction** (R), which can be combined with side-to-side movements to produce a circular **grinding movement** between the molars.

All these movements have mobile axes and are typical of movements taking place around **instantaneous and changing axes,** as is the rule in biomechanics.

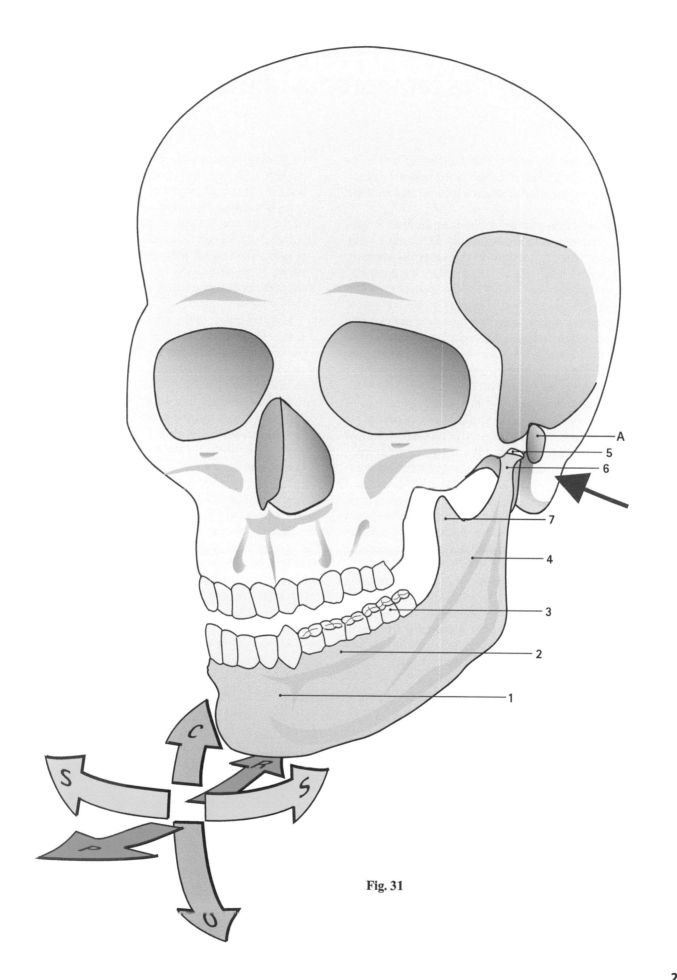

Fig. 31

The structure of the temporomandibular joint

The **temporomandibular joint** (Fig. 32) consists of two articular surfaces: a superior surface attached to the inferior surface of the basicranium and an inferior surface located on top of the mandibular ramus.

- The **superior articular surface** is the **mandibular or glenoid fossa** concave in both directions but particularly anteriorly. It lies inferior and anterior to the **external acoustic meatus** (A), whose inferior wall is formed by the tympanic part of the **temporal bone** (1). This fossa is continuous anteriorly with the **posterior surface** (2) of the transverse root of the anteroposteriorly convex **zygomatic process** (3), which gives rise to the **articular tubercle.** The bottom of this fossa is traversed from side to side by the **petrotympanic or Glaserian fossa** (4), *lying between the tympanic part* (T) *of the temporal bone posteriorly and the zygomatic process anteriorly.* The **anterior part** (the preglaserian part) (2) of the mandibular fossa **is articular and lined by cartilage**; its **posterior part** (the retroglaserian part) is **non-articular.** On the other hand, the cartilage lining the anterior part extends over *the surface of the articular tubercle*, which is **also articular.** Thus this articular surface is **concave posteriorly and convex anteriorly.**

- The **inferior articular surface** is a cartilage-coated ovoid surface splayed out transversely, i.e. the **condylar process** supported by the neck of the mandible (N). The process is shown here in two positions: 1) when the mouth is closed (C), it lies within the **glenoid fossa**; 2) when the mouth is open (O), it rests on the most prominent part of the articular tubercle.

- The **articular disc** (6) is *located between the two articular surfaces.* It is a supple and flexible **biconcave** fibrocartilaginous structure, which is *mobile relative to the two surfaces* and follows the movements of the condylar process by gliding inside the joint cavity. It is shown here in two positions, i.e. with the mouth closed (5) and with the mouth open (6). It is held in check by the **upper lamina** (7), which is a **restraining ligament** running from the tympanic part of the temporal bone to its posterior border. When this ligament is stretched (8), the disc is pulled back during mouth closure. The **lateral pterygoid** (9) is inserted into the neck of the condylar process and also by an expansion (10) into the anterior border of the disc, which pulls the disc forwards during mouth closure.

- The anterior part of the **articular capsule** is attached to the disc (11), while its posterior part (12) connects the tympanic part of the temporal bone directly to the neck of the condylar process.

Simplistically one could imagine the convex condylar process rotating in the mandibular fossa around an axis located in the centre of the fossa, but the reality is *quite different.*

- **During mouth opening** (Fig. 33) the condylar process moves anteriorly on the posterior surface of the articular tubercle without overshooting its crest (black arrow).

- A lateral view (Fig. 34) of the **movement of mouth opening** shows that its mobile axis **O** lies somewhere below the joint at the level of the **mandibular** lingula visible on the inner surface of the ramus.

The very unusual functional anatomy of the joint explains why *it is difficult to reduce temporomandibular dislocations* when the **condylar process has overstepped the crest of the articular tubercle.** It can only be brought back by **strongly pulling down the posterior part of the mandible** so that its condylar process can then be pushed back into position; this is achieved by placing both thumbs on the patient's most posterior inferior molars and applying pressure downwards (blue arrow).

Fig. 32

Fig. 33

Fig. 34

The movements of the temporomandibular joint

In joints with such complex movements the axes can only be defined by analysing the elementary movements. This joint has five types of movement taking place around the following axes (Fig. 35):

- a horizontal axis (xx') for movements involved in opening and closing the mouth (Fig. 36) occurring between xx' and yy'; it is not the condyle but the entire mandible that slides anteriorly
- the plane for anteroposterior translation of the mandible, i.e. protrusion and retraction (Fig. 37), whose axis (as we have already seen, p. 296) lies very far down at the level of the mandibular lingula
- an axis for side-to-side sliding movements when the entire mandible moves (Fig. 38)
- an axis for vertical rotation (v) occurring in either joint during lateral movements (Fig. 39); one of the two condylar processes stays put in the mandibular fossa and acts as a pivot while the other slides anteriorly on the anterior surface of the glenoid fossa
- an oblique axis (u) located in either joint for eccentric jaw opening, i.e. jaw opening combined with lateral movement (Fig. 40). This combined movement is the most difficult to perform, since it combines opening of the mouth and a vertical rotation. Excessive opening of the mouth as during yawning can drag the two condylar processes beyond the edge of the articular tubercle. The condyles become stuck and the dislocation becomes permanent and irreducible, requiring an operative intervention for reduction.

All these movements can be combined with tangential shearing movements, which are needed to crush very hard pieces of food.

Fig. 35

Fig. 36

Fig. 37

Fig. 38

Fig. 39

Fig. 40

Muscles of jaw closure

There are **three** muscles controlling jaw closure, with two of them visible on a **lateral view of the skull** (Fig. 41):

- the **temporalis** (1), which is a wide, flat, powerful muscle arising fanwise from the entire surface of the temporal fossa above the zygomatic process; its tendon passes deep to the zygomatic process before its insertion into the coronoid process of the mandible
- the **masseter** (2) arising from the inferior border of the zygomatic arch and inserted into the lateral surface of the angle of the mandible
- the **medial pterygoid** (3), which arises from the concave medial surface of the **pterygoid process** (5) and is directed obliquely inferiorly and medially to be inserted into the *medial surface* of the angle of the mandible. As a result, this third muscle is visible only after one half of the opposite mandible has been resected. This **lateral view of the skull** (Fig. 42) *shows the medial surface of the right mandible* after resection of the left mandible.

These two figures show clearly that these three muscles *strongly pull the angle of the mandible upwards*. The fact that some acrobats can remain suspended by their jaws attests to the power of these muscles.

Figure 43 is a posterior view of the mandible, which is slightly asymmetrical and tilted to the right to display the posterior surface of the mandible, the pterygoid plate (5) and the zygomatic arch (6) with these three muscles:

- the **temporalis** (1) running upwards between the coronoid process and the temporal fossa
- the **masseter** (2) lying laterally and arising above from the zygomatic process (6)
- the **medial pterygoid** (3) lying medially and arising from the pterygoid process (5); it acts as a muscular 'hammock' to elevate the angle of the mandible.

Also visible is the **lateral pterygoid** (4) running transversely from the lateral surface of the **pterygoid process** (5) to the neck of the mandibular condyle. This muscle does not elevate the mandible but participates in jaw opening (see p. 303).

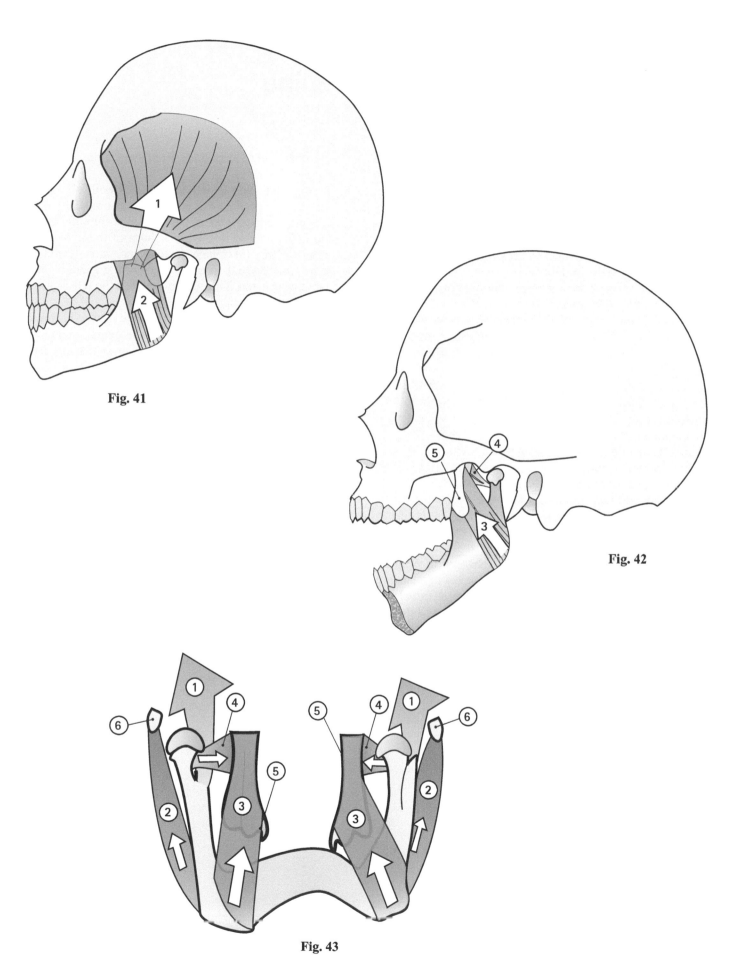

Fig. 41

Fig. 42

Fig. 43

The muscles involved in jaw opening

These muscles are more numerous and less powerful than those for jaw closing. It is worth noting at the outset that gravity favours jaw opening, as happens during sleep or after loss of consciousness. *All but one of the muscles are located below the mandible.* **The hyoid bone and the thyroid cartilage** act as relay stations between the mandible and the superior thoracic inlet, which is formed by the *first ribs* on both sides and the *manubrium sterni* in the middle.

These muscles fall into **two groups**: the suprahyoid and the infrahyoid muscles (Fig. 44).

The **infrahyoid muscles** connect the **thyrohyoid complex** to the *shoulder girdle and the sternum.* At the inferior border of the hyoid bone (h) they are the following mediolaterally:

- The **thyrohyoid** (1) runs vertically from the hyoid bone to be inserted into the oblique line of the thyroid cartilage (t), and it is continuous inferiorly with the **sternothyroid** (2) running from the margin of the oblique line of the thyroid to the manubrium.
- The **sternohyoid** (3) extends from its manubrial origin lateral to the sternothyroid and from the medial extremity of the clavicle to its insertion into the hyoid bone.
- The **omohyoid** is a thin *digastric* muscle arising from the superior border of the scapula. Its inferior belly (4) is directed superiorly, medially and laterally to end in the **intermediate tendon** at the level of the supraclavicular fossa. From this point onwards its superior belly (5) changes direction to ascend almost vertically before being inserted into the inferior border of the hyoid, lateral to the first three muscles.

All these infrahyoid muscles **lower the hyoid bone and the thyroid cartilage** and resist the action of the suprahyoid muscles. The **suprahyoid muscles** constitute the upper storey of muscles involved in jaw opening.

The hyoid bone is attached posteriorly to the basicranium by the following muscles:

- the **stylohyoid** (6) running from the *styloid process* (s) to the hyoid bone
- the **digastric** muscle, whose **posterior belly** (7) arises from the mastoid process (m) and runs inferomedially to end in the intermediate tendon, which passes through its **fibrous loop** (8) attached to the lesser horn of the hyoid bone; its **anterior belly** (9) changes direction and runs superomedially to be attached to the inner surface of the mandible near the symphysis menti. The anterior belly of the left digastric (9′) is also visible in the diagram.

The hyoid bone is attached to the mandible by two other muscles:

- The **geniohyoid** (10) arises from the genial tubercle on the inner surface of the mandible and is inserted into the hyoid bone.
- The **mylohyoid** (11) is a wide, flat, triangular muscle with the shape of a half paper cone; it arises from the inner surface of the mandible to be inserted into the hyoid bone. The two mylohyoids form the **floor of the mouth.**

All these suprahyoid muscles **lower the mandible** when they **act from the hyoid bone**, which is *kept fixed by the infrahyoid muscles.* We have already seen that the suprahyoids are **remote flexors of the cervical spine** when they act in concert with the muscles of mastication.

The last muscle concerned with jaw opening is the **lateral pterygoid**, visible on a **medial view of the mandible below the basicranium** (Fig. 45). Its fleshy fibres (12) arise from the external surface of the pterygoid process (a) and are inserted into the anterior aspect of the neck of the condylar process (c). It *pulls the condylar neck anteriorly*, and in so doing it *tilts the mandible* around its centre of rotation O, causing the mouth to open. Without this action the *condylar process would remain jammed in the mandibular fossa.* It also **pulls the articular disc anteriorly** (see Fig. 32, p. 297). Thus the lateral pterygoid plays an essential role in jaw opening.

s

6

m

9'

10

9

11

7

8

h

1

t

3

5

2

4

Fig. 44

c 12 a

O

Fig. 45

The role of muscles in mandibular movements

It is now possible to relate movements of the mandible to the actions of specific muscles.

- **Protrusion** (Fig. 46), i.e. forward movement of the mandible, is produced by the simultaneous contraction of the **two lateral pterygoids.**
- **Lateral translation without pericondylar rotation** (Fig. 47, black arrows) is produced by contraction of the **contralateral lateral pterygoid** and of the **ipsilateral masseter** (not shown in the diagram).
- **Side-to-side movement without lateral translation or pericondylar rotation** (Fig. 48) is produced by the *ipsilateral* **masseter** and the *contralateral* **medial pterygoid.**
- **Side-to-side movement around an oblique axis** at one of the temporomandibular joints (Fig. 49) is produced by the simultaneous contraction of the *ipsilateral* **masseter** and the *contralateral* **lateral pterygoid.**
- Lowering of the mandible and **jaw opening** (Fig. 50) are brought about by the simultaneous contraction of the **supra- and infrahyoid muscles** and of the **lateral pterygoids.**
- Finally, **jaw closure** (Fig. 51) and occlusion of the teeth are produced by simultaneous bilateral contraction of the muscles of mastication, i.e. the **temporals**, the **masseters** and the **medial pterygoids.**

During mastication in real life all these elementary muscle actions are combined in various proportions and strengths, which change during the performance of the movement.

Fig. 46

Fig. 47

Fig. 48

Fig. 49

Fig. 50

Fig. 51

305

The eyeball: a perfect enarthrosis

Orthopaedic surgeons and physiotherapists do not realize that the eyeball is an **enarthrosis**, a *spheroidal joint like the hip or the shoulder*. It is indeed a **perfect enarthrosis** (Fig. 52: section of the orbit) with a spherical globe formed by the pliable but resistant *sclera* (1), which is flanked externally by *the fascial sheath of the eyeball* (2) (Tenon's capsule). The *intervening episcleral space* or Tenon's space (3) forms a gliding surface, which is spherical, flexible and permanently adaptable and accommodates more than 50% of the globe – more than usual in enarthroses. The fascial sheath of the eyeball is *thick around the equator* (2) and becomes progressively *thinner and more flexible* (4) towards the poles, particularly the **posterior pole** (5), which is pierced by the optic nerve (6).

This spherical structure is surrounded by the semi-fluid *orbital fat pad* (7) and is attached to the walls of the orbit by the *check ligaments* (8) of the eyeball arising from the sheaths (9) of the ocular muscles, i.e. the **superior rectus** (10), the **inferior rectus** (11), the **inferior oblique** (12, seen in cross-section) and the **levator palpebrae** (13). (The other ocular muscles are not visible in this diagram.) It is the best elastic *suspension system in the body*. It is *perfectly protected* **inside the bony wall of the orbit** (14) by the anteriorly located **lids** (15), and it is covered by the conjunctiva, which is reflected on the eyeball to form the **conjunctival fornix** (16).

This enarthrosis is so perfect that it could be *taken as the paragon* for enarthroses. It comprises **three muscle pairs**, *one for each degree of freedom*.
- The two pairs of **rectus muscles** (Fig. 53) are responsible for **horizontal and vertical eye movements**, as follows:
  - *upward*: **superior rectus** (sr)
  - *downward*: **inferior rectus** (ir)
  - *side-to-side*: **lateral rectus** (lr) for the same direction as the gaze; **medial rectus** (mr) for the opposite side.

For a **horizontal or vertical gaze** the spheroidal joint of the eyeball simply behaves like a **universal joint** with *two axes* (one vertical and the other horizontal) and *two degrees of freedom*.

- The process is more complicated when the **gaze is oblique** (Fig. 54) either upwards or downwards. Then a third pair of *muscles* is recruited, i.e. the **two rotator muscles** acting in symmetrically opposite fashion around the polar anteroposterior axis (p), orthogonal to both the vertical (v) and the horizontal (h) axes, as follows:
  - The **inferior oblique** (io) is the simpler of the two. It is attached to the lateral surface of the eyeball, *skirts round its equator from below* and then runs medially to gain attachment to the inferomedial angle of the orbit. The **left inferior oblique** turns the eyeball **clockwise**; the **right inferior oblique** turns it **anticlockwise**. They are thus *perfect antagonists* and never contract *simultaneously*.
  - The **superior oblique** is a more complex muscle. It is a *digastric muscle* with its *intermediate tendon* being reflected in a *fibrous pulley* attached to the superomedial angle of the orbit. Its first belly follows the same path as the inferior oblique but in the opposite direction; from its attachment to the lateral surface of the eyeball it *skirts around its equator from above* and is directed medially to reach its pulley. From there the second belly *changes direction* to gain attachment to the roof of the orbit along with the rectus muscles. The **left superior oblique** (lso) turns the eyeball *anticlockwise* and the **right superior oblique** (rso) turns it *clockwise*. They are thus *perfect antagonists* and never contract *simultaneously*. On the other hand, they enjoy a **crossed synergy** with the inferior obliques, i.e. the right superior oblique is synergistic with the left inferior oblique and vice versa. Likewise, they are **ipsilateral antagonists**, i.e. the *right superior oblique antagonizes the right inferior oblique and similarly on the left*.

Fig. 52

Fig. 53

Fig. 54

The ocular muscles in horizontal and vertical eye movements

Horizontal and vertical movements of the eyeballs are easy to explain by simply looking at the actions of the recti:

For **horizontal side-to-side glances** (Fig. 55) the medial and lateral recti contract as follows:

- for a **glance to the right** the right lateral rectus and the left medial rectus contract at the same time to rotate the eyeball on its vertical axis (v)
- for a **glance to the left** the converse is true, with simultaneous contraction of the left lateral rectus and right medial rectus.

For **vertical glances** (Fig. 56) the superior and inferior rectus muscles contract:

- for the **upward glance** both superior recti rotate the eyeball on its horizontal axis (h)
- for the **downward glance** the converse is true, with contraction of both inferior recti.

During these two types of movement the spheroidal joint of the eyeball **behaves mechanically like a universal joint**, i.e. like a joint with two axes and two degrees of freedom. The third degree of freedom, i.e. rotation of the eyeball on its polar axis (e) is not utilized, and it is not shown.

Fig. 55

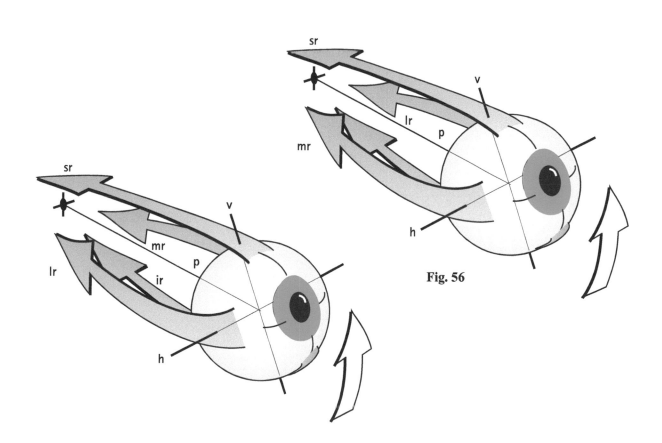

Fig. 56

The ocular muscles in eye convergence

Stereovision (Fig. 57) requires **convergence of the eyes** so that the images received by both eyes are as identical as possible. The nearest point of convergence for both eyes is called the **punctum proximum** (PP).

A very distant object on the horizon or in the sky lies beyond the **far point** or **punctum remotum** (PR), which represents the limit for convergence of the eyes. At this point there is no **parallax** and the *images in both eyes are identical*; *the sense of depth disappears* and *distance can no longer be estimated with any precision*. **Telemetry** (the intuitive measurement of distance) therefore depends critically on the degree of convergence of the visual axes of both eyes.

For the far point the rays are **almost parallel**, i.e. *without any parallax*. But, if for instance the base B (i.e. the **interpupillary distance**) is doubled, the far point will recede by a factor of two compared with the normal base. *Gunners*, particularly in the *navy*, used this **telemetric principle** to evaluate the distance of their target, and the width of the gun turret served as a base. This method is now out of date with the **use of radar** but the principle is still valid.

Likewise, stereovision is only possible if **both eyes face forwards**, which is not the case with most birds, except the **birds of prey** (like the eagle), which can thus locate their prey with great precision. One can conclude that *predators need to have eyes that face forwards!*

What happens **within the range of the far point**? Distance depends on the angle of convergence (p) and is estimated as the **difference in tension between the two medial recti** (mr)

until the **near point (punctum proximum [PP])** is reached, when convergence is lost. Thus, within this range, the difference between the *two images becomes progressively greater as the object gets closer*, and this produces the **sensation of depth** in the cerebral cortex.

The extremely rapid computation of the **instantaneous distance** of a **moving object**, which therefore represents a threat, is carried out in the **brainstem.** Let us imagine this process in action in tennis players who see the ball coming their way at great speed and must estimate its speed and predict its trajectory. This is a tribute to **our marvellous computer** but it also explains why tennis players do not last long in their careers: a tennis player must not only imagine the trajectory of the ball but also **in a fraction of a second** determine how to move the arm holding the racquet and choose a body orientation so as to intercept the ball and send it back in a direction unforeseen by the opponent. Once again, what a marvellous performance!

In the normal subject, the convergence of the axes of both eyes is controlled *perfectly and automatically* by the nervous system and the contraction of the ocular muscles, in particular the medial and lateral recti. Failure of this mechanism of control leads to **strabismus**, which is of the internal type when the axes are too convergent and of the external type when the axes are divergent. This disorder can have a neurological or a muscular cause, e.g. when the recti are either too short or too long, as is the case in *congenital strabismus*, which can be corrected by *surgery* on one of the lateral recti.

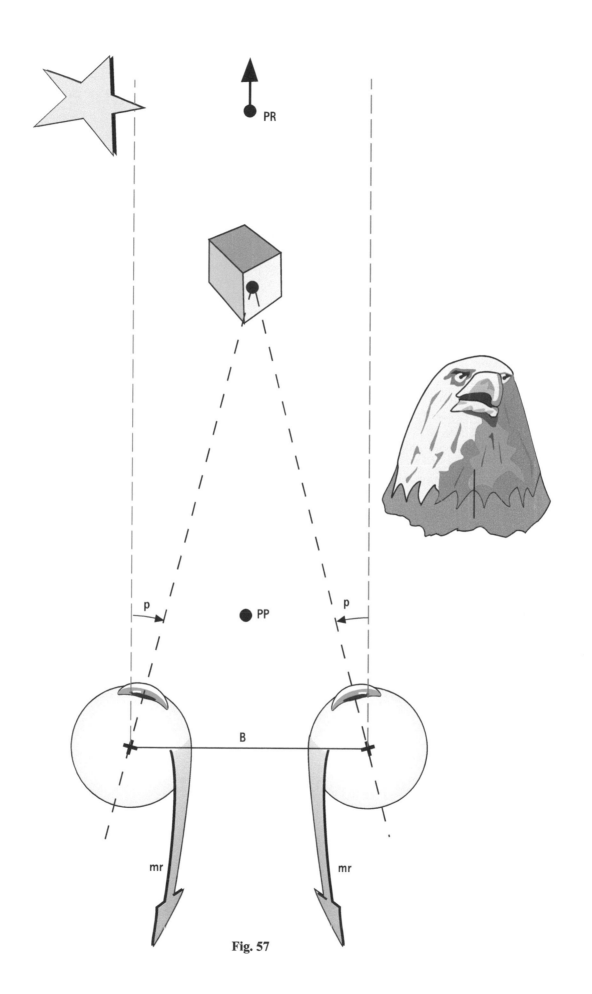

Fig. 57

The mechanical problem of the oblique glance

Horizontal and vertical eye movements are easily understood, but understanding eye movements during **oblique glances** poses a problem, which can be solved by reverting to the notion of the **universal joint** discussed in Volume 1 in relation to the shoulder (Codman's paradox, p. 18) and the trapezometacarpal joint (rotation into pronation of the pillar of the thumb, p. 266). In the **position of rest** (Fig. 58), i.e. the eyes looking straight ahead towards the horizon, the horizontal meridian **m** of the eyeball is *parallel to the horizon.* It is represented by the line **k** in the *model of the universal joint* (Fig. 59).

When the **eyes are lowered** (Fig. 60), the meridian **m** stays *parallel* to the line representing the horizontal (k) in the model, which performs the same movement around the axis **h** (Fig. 61). If the eyes, already lowered, are moved **to the right** (Fig. 62), the meridian **m** is no longer horizontal and is now *tilted obliquely downwards and to the left.* This change is illustrated by the model of the universal joint (Fig. 63), where the mobile segment rotates on both axes and undergoes an **automatic rotation** or **conjunct rotation** (MacConnail) on its long axis, in accordance with the mechanical properties of a universal joint. As a result, the *horizon is no longer horizontal.*

At this point a corrective counter-rotation occurs (Fig. 64), as is possible in a joint with **three degrees of freedom**, i.e. an enarthrosis. This **reflex rotation** is produced in this case by *contraction of the muscle that surrounds the eyeball from above,* i.e. the **inferior oblique** (io), which brings back the meridian **m** to the horizontal position so that the *horizon will appear horizontal in the image provided by this eye.* In the model (Fig. 65) a third corrective rotation takes place as line k moves to position k', i.e. back into the horizontal plane. This corrective conjunct rotation is produced by contraction of the superior oblique (so) and the inferior oblique (io); it is *entirely reflex and of central origin* and is the result of an extremely precise mechanism. The efferent messages are carried by the oculomotor nerve (the third cranial nerve) to the inferior oblique (io) and by the trochlear nerve (the fourth cranial nerve) to the superior oblique (so).

This is the *same mechanism* that corrects the **pseudoparadox of Codman at the shoulder** (see Volume 1, p. 19). Likewise, it is the **conjunct rotation** in the trapezometacarpal joint (a universal joint) that **rotates the thumb into pronation during opposition** (see Volume 1, p. 303).

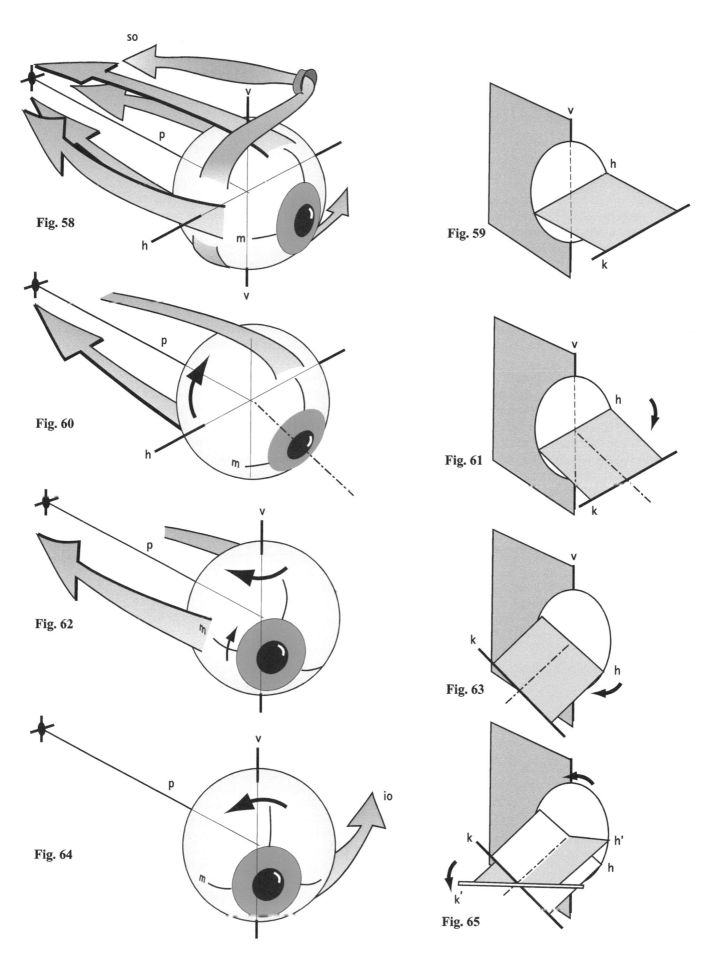

Fig. 58

Fig. 59

Fig. 60

Fig. 61

Fig. 62

Fig. 63

Fig. 64

Fig. 65

The oblique glance: the role of the oblique muscles and of the trochlear nerve

The importance of the third degree of freedom in the control of the movements of the ocular muscles is now apparent, making it possible to describe these movements during oblique glances. When the **glance is oblique upwards** (Fig. 66), expressing **fear, consternation** or **despair** (as does the 'tearful sister', who *looks upwards and to the right* in the painting *The Prodigal Son* by J-B Greuze, Louvre Museum), the horizontal planes tilt *downwards and to the right* (Fig. 67). This obliquely directed component (o) is corrected by contraction of the **superior oblique on the right side** (so) and the **inferior oblique on the left side** (io). The coordinated and simultaneous contraction of these muscles brings back the meridian **r** to coincide with the horizontal plane for the image provided by each eye.

When the **glance is oblique downwards and to the left** (Fig. 68), expressing disdain or irony (as in the painting *The Bohemian* by F. Hals, Louvre Museum), the horizontal planes tilt downwards and to the left (Fig. 69), and the image is righted by contraction of the left superior oblique (so) and of the right inferior oblique (io). This coordinated and simultaneous contraction of these two muscles brings back the meridian **r** to coincide with the horizontal plane for the image provided by each eye.

The usefulness of these two small muscles is now obvious, although it tends to escape the notice of a novice in anatomy. They correct automatically the conjunct rotation produced by the oblique glance.

The marvellous aspect of this mechanism lies in the fact that *two different muscles innervated by two different nerves act simultaneously and in perfect harmony* in order to correct precisely an unwanted rotational component and thus **reestablish the coincidence of horizontal and vertical planes.** Without this correction the two slightly different images could not be interpreted in **stereovision.**

The **trochlear nerve**, the *fourth cranial nerve*, was formerly known as the *pathetic nerve* because of its role in expressing the pathetic look. It is purely motor and *innervates a single muscle*, the **superior oblique.** Patients suffering from a transient virally induced paralysis of this nerve are aware that they cannot bring into line both horizontal planes, a major impediment in driving. The **inferior oblique** is innervated by the **oculomotor nerve** (*the third cranial nerve*), which innervates all the ocular muscles except the **lateral rectus**, which is innervated by a single nerve, the **abducens nerve** (*the sixth cranial nerve*).

Fig. 66

Fig. 68

Fig. 67

Fig. 69

APPENDICES

Mass, weight and barycentres

Weight and **mass** are often confused, but they are different, albeit related, ideas. The mass of an object corresponds to the quantity of matter it contains, i.e., the sum total of all its molecules. The unit of **mass** is the kilogram (kg), and its value is the same, wherever the object happens to be in the universe: for example, the mass of an astronaut is identical on whatever planet he happens to be (Fig. 1. M. E and J). **Weight** is a *measure of the attractive force* exerted on the object by the planet on which it lies. Its unit is the **Newton** (N) from the name of the scientist who discovered the 'law of universal attraction'. This force varies according to the planet of residence: in the case of the astronaut, he weighs less (his weight is shown as the arrow pointing downwards) on the moon (M) than on Earth (E) or on Jupiter (J) in accordance with the **force of gravity** (g). Thus on Earth g is equal to 9.8 N/kg, but on the Moon it is only 1.6 N/kg; hence his weight on the Moon is only 1/6 of his weight on earth. In contrast, on Jupiter, the largest of the planets in the Solar System, where g equals 24.8 N/kg, his weight will be equal to two and one half times his weight on Earth and he will have difficulty in moving. In the spacecraft, however, his weight is zero, since he is in a **weightless** (no gravity) environment, but his whole mass is conserved, since a certain force is needed to displace him and overcome his inertia.

To perform calculations in mechanics it is assumed that all the mass in a body is concentrated in a virtual point, called the **barycentre** (formerly known as 'the centre of gravity'). The problem is localising this point, which is **totally fictitious** but nonetheless very real.

On a flat surface the answer is relatively simple. For a triangle (Fig. 2) it lies at the point of intersection of its three medians; for a circle it lies at the centre.

In space, if one realises that the barycentre always lies on the vertical line running through the site where the object is suspended, then one can easily localise it by suspending the object at multiple sites of attachment. For example, for a cardboard triangle it lies at the point of intersection of its medians (Fig. 2); for a sphere (Fig. 4) at its centre; for a tetrahedron as shown in Fig. 3, and even for a pear as shown in Fig. 5.

Suppose now that we are looking at the barycentre of a dumbbell with two unequal masses (Fig. 6). Logically it will lie on the bar of the dumbbell, but where? The answer is that it lies **much closer to the heavier mass** at a point O so that AO/OB is **inversely proportional to W_1/W_2**. One can easily 'construct' this point as follows:

- Apply to point A (the barycentre of the heavier mass S_1) the weight vector W_2 of the smaller mass S_2 **in an upward direction** in order to obtain the point w'_2
- Apply to the barycentre B of the smaller mass S_2 the downward vector p_1, which represents the weight vector W_1 of the mass S_1 and extends to the point w_1
- Draw a straight line to join w_1 to w'_2
- This line will intersect the bar of the dumbbell at **O**, which represents the barycentre of the dumbbell with unequal masses and also the point where the dumbbell can be perfectly balanced and where the combined weight $W_1 + W_2$ is applied.

When there are multiple bodies – e.g., three, as in figure 7 – simply 'construct' in the same way the barycentre **O'** between the bodies **A** and **B**, then that of **O''** between **A** and **C**, and finally the common barycentre **O'''**, where the combined weight $W_1 + W_2 + W_3 = R$ is applied.

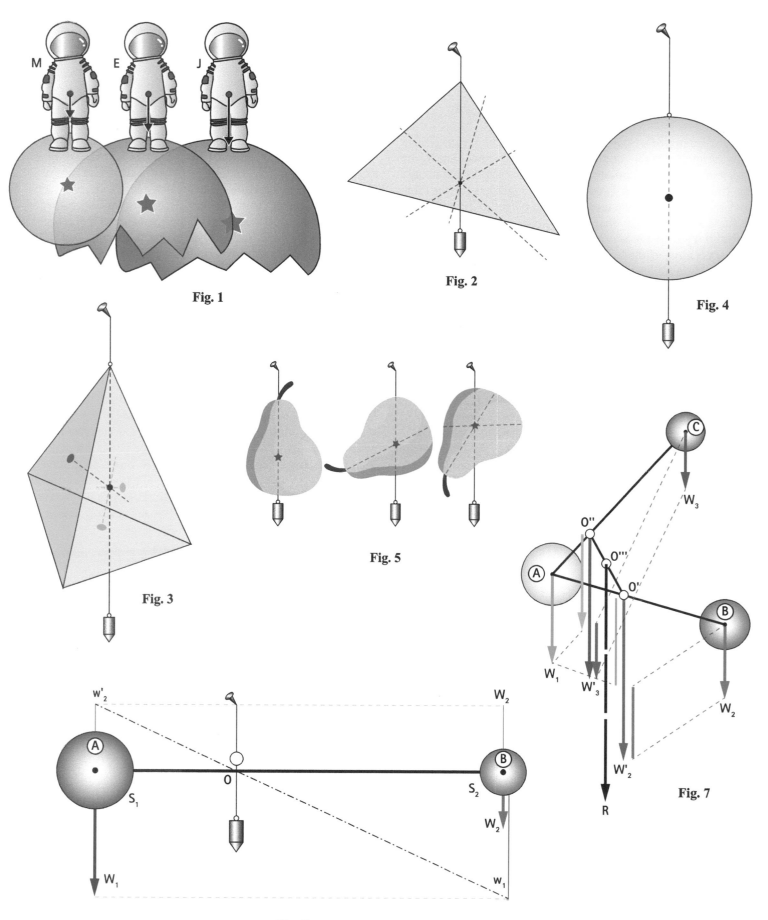

Fig. 1

Fig. 2

Fig. 3

Fig. 4

Fig. 5

Fig. 6

Fig. 7

How to localise barycentres

The barycentre of a body is only fixed or unchangeable if that body is unchangeable and undeformable. The position of the barycentre of the **astronaut** (Fig. 8) has been determined only to a first approximation, because he is thought to keep the same posture regardless of the identity of the planet of his choice.

In fact, a living body changes its shape constantly, and its **global barycentre** moves according to the location of the partial barycentres of the segments of its limbs. Figure 9 shows a man standing still with the partial barycentres of each of the segments of his limbs clearly identified. In his upper limb can be seen the barycentres of the forearm **A** and of the arm **B**, which combine to form the barycentre of the upper limb **S**. Likewise the segmental barycentres of the lower limbs **C** and J combine to form the partial barycentre of the lower limb **I**. The two segmental barycentres of the lower limbs combine to form the global barycentre of the lower limbs **MI** (star), and those of the upper limbs combine to form the global barycentres of the upper limbs **MS** (star). Similarly, the barycentres of head and neck **TC** and that of the thorax combine to form the partial barycentre **TT** (square). Combining the barycentres of the upper and lower limbs gives the barycentre of the four limbs **M**. Finally, by combining the barycentres **M** and **TT**, one obtains the **global barycentre G** of the body of this man standing still. It is located in the pelvis at the level S3, midway between the sacral promontory and the pubis both in the man (Fig. 9) and in the woman (Fig. 10).

Let us now determine the global barycentres of some people in motion. For a woman sitting cross-legged with her lower limbs folded, her global barycentre (red star) is displaced upwards along her abdomen and comes to lie above the umbilicus. In the case of the **running jumper** (Fig. 12), her **global barycentre** is displaced forwards by the forward projection of her upper limbs. For the **fast walker** (Fig. 13) her global barycentre oscillates forwards and backwards because of the vigorous swinging of her upper limbs. In these cases the global barycentre stays 'inside the body', but it can come to lie 'outside the body' in some cases when the body is bent. Thus, **when one climbs on all fours** (Fig. 14), the global barycentre is located clearly anterior to the trunk, and **when one jumps with the trunk hyperextended** (Fig. 15), the global barycentre tends to come to lie posterior to the body. This method of localising the **global barycentre** can be used for all daily activites, e.g., while working or doing sports, especially **figure skating** (Fig. 16), when one realises that to keep the *force vector starting from R along the blade of the skate*, the skater's brain must retain without fail the routines needed for balance in order to avoid falling on the ice or on the podium. This is necessary because the resultant **R** varies continuously due to the fact that the centrifugal force **C** has a circular trajectory and combines with the body weight **P**. Hence the need for daily practice.

Fig. 8

Fig. 9

Fig. 10

Fig. 11

Fig. 12

Fig. 13

Fig. 14

Fig. 15

Fig. 16

T.C

B

S

M.S

T.T

Tr

A

G

M

C

I

M.I

J

C

R

P

t

321

Joint hypermobility

Some individuals (particularly Asian) seen at fairs or circuses and on television enjoy absolutely extraordinary ranges of joint movements as a result of **hyperlaxity of their ligaments**, which they develop further from very early in life but at the cost of many years of daily training and exercise approaching physical torture. It is the **spinal column** that receives particular training, especially *in extension*, because flexion is quite soon limited by the presence of the abdomen.

The basic exercise is **doing 'the crab' in extension** (Fig. 17), allowing the hands to reach the ground and even the ankles. Measurement of this extension from the previously established plane of the superior surface of the first sacral vertebra (also called the *sacral plateau*) to the previously established plane of the bite reveals a range of 205°, vastly exceeding the 140° range of extension of the normal spinal column (see p. 39).

In this position of doing 'the crab', some individuals can bring their heads to touch their buttocks (Fig. 18), corresponding to an extension of 240°. It must be stressed that this hyperextension **takes place only in the lumbar and more so in the cervical segment of the spinal column**. In fact the thoracic segment is much less flexible in flexion-extension because of the presence of the thoracic cage. The most talented of these individuals can even surpass this degree of extension and can bring the **nape of the neck in front of the buttocks** (Fig. 19).

This hyperlaxity is usually seen in females, since they are more flexible than males. It can also be associated with the **Ehlers-Danloss syndrome**, a congenital defect of the connective tissues. As regards their joints, it is quite commonplace to see women able to turn their thumbs to face the other way. At any rate, classical ballerinas can do the splits more easily than men, and a star performer can raise her left lower limb straight up while standing on the tip of her right foot.

All these physical exercises are *typical of humans*, always haunted by the desire to better their achievements. No zoologist has ever mentioned seeing an orangutan doing 'the crab'. If it were possible it would have been known since Cuvier's time. Some monkeys, especially chimpanzees, are able to smile, gainsaying Rabelais's statement that 'smiling is the property of the human being'.

205°

Fig. 17

240°

Fig. 18

Fig. 19

The law of parsimony: Occam's razor

Nature oscillates between two extremes corresponding to two important laws: **the law of parsimony and the law of profusion**. The first law, **the law of parsimony**, has been established by William of Ockham (1290-1349), an English monk and philosopher, who died after being excommunicated. This law stipulates that 'all that is unnecessary should be discarded'; hence its name of **Occam's razor**. This law, which appeals to reason, has many applications in Nature, especially in the musculoskeletal system. In Nature, it is perfectly illustrated by the sphere (Fig. 20) , which has the maximum for the minimum surface. The egg (Fig. 21) is another example: the minimum amount of shell protects the maximum volume for the embryo. The mechanical resistance of the sphere or of an ovoid is maximal when compared with that of other structures; for example, the ovoid cranium (Fig. 22) can hold the maximal amount of cerebral tissue inside a container of minimal surface area and of maximal resistance. The cerebral convolutions also illustrate the theory of fractals, which can be deemed to be an application of the law of parsimony: to lodge the maximal amount of cortical surface in the minimal volume. The second law, called **the law of profusion** is valid in the domain of **large numbers**, typically concerned with **reproduction** and **natural selection** and illustrated here diagrammatically. Figure 23 shows the competition among millions of spermatozoa as they approach the ovum with only one achieving success, just like the thousands of sea turtles hatched on the shore and desperately trying to reach the sea before falling prey to predatory birds. Figure 24 shows shoals of fish, as thick as clouds, trying to escape and breaking ranks before being caught by their predators. Finally, witness the millions of grains of pollen scattered by the wind for only one to reach the pistil of a flower.

Why such an apparent waste? Because in the case of **natural selection** the lottery of large numbers must operate in choosing the luckiest or the fittest, Nature appears cruel with her **implacable logic**.

Fig. 20

Fig. 21

Fig. 22

Fig. 23

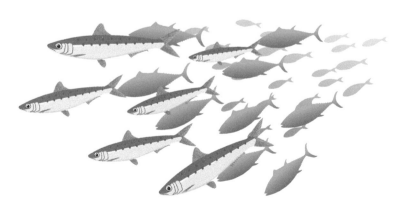

Fig. 24

Bibliography

Azerad J 1992 *Physiologie de la manducation.* Masson, Paris

Barnett CH, Davies DV, MacConaill MA 1961 *Synovial joints. Their structure and mechanics.* C.C. Thomas, Springfield

Barnier L 1950 *L'analyse des mouvements.* PUF, Paris

Basmajian JV 1962 *Muscles alive. Their function revealed by electromyography.* Williams & Wilkins, Baltimore

Bouisset S 2002 *Biomécanique et physiologie du mouvement.* Masson, Paris

Bridgeman GB 1939 *The human machine. The anatomical structure and mechanism of the human body*, Vol. 1. Dover Publications, New York

Brinckmann P, Frobin W, Leivseth G 2002 *Musculoskeletal biomechanics.* Thième, New York

Bunnell S 1970 *Surgery of the hand*, 5th edn revised by Boyes. Lippincott, Philadelphia (1st edn. 1944)

Calais-Germain B 1984 *Anatomie du mouvement*, Vol. 1. Désiris, Revel

Calais-Germain B 2005 *Anatomie du mouvement. Bases d'exercices.* Désiris, Revel

Cardano, Gerolamo (Italian mathematician 1501-1576) À propos du cardan: see the Internet

Duchenne (de Boulogne) GBA 1867 *Physiologie des mouvements 1.* J.-B. Baillière, Paris (out of print; edited facsimile published by Annales de Médecine Physique, 1967)

Duchenne (de Boulogne) GBA 1949 *Physiology of motion.* Translated by E.B. Kaplan. W.B. Saunders, Philadelphia

Esnault M 2005 *Rachis et stretching* Masson, Paris

Feher G, Szunyoghy A 1996 *Grand cours d'anatomie artistique.* Könemann, Köln

Fischer O 1907 *Kinematik orhanischer Gelenke.* F. Vierweg, Braunsschweig

Gasquet (de) B 1997 *Bien-être et maternité.* Implexe éditions, Paris

Gauss, Karl Friedrich (German mathematician, 1777-1855) *La géométrie non euclidienne* (on Codman's paradox): see the Internet

Ghyka MC 1978 *Le Nombre d'or.* Gallimard, Paris

Goudot R, Hérisson C 2003 *Pathologie de l'articulation temporomandibulaire.* Masson, Paris

Hamonet C., Brissot R., Anne Gompel A. et al. (Faculté de Médecine de Créteil). 'Ehlers-Danlos Syndrome (EDS) – Contribution to Clinical Diagnosis – A Prospective Study of 853 Patients'. *EC Neurology*, 10.6 (2018) : 428-439.

Heimlich HJ La manœuvre d'Heimlich. Online. Available: www.heimlichinstitute.org

Henke J 1859 Die Bewegungen der Hanwurzel. *Zeitschrift für rationelle Medizine* 7:27

Henke W 1863 *Handbuch der Anatomie und Mechanik der Gelenke.* C.F. Wintersche, Heidelberg

Kapandji AI 1987 La Biomécanique patate. *Ann Chir Main* 5:260-263

Kapandji AI 1997 Vous avez dit Biomécanique? La Mécanique 'floue' ou 'patate'. *Maîtrise Orthopédique* 64:1-11

Kapandji A.I. Qu'est-ce que la biomécanique? Éditions Sauramps Médical, Montpellier, 2011.

Lievre JA, Bloch-Michel H, Attali P 1957 Trans-sacral injection: clinical and radiological study. *Bull Mem Soc Med Hop Paris* 73(33-34):1110-1118

MacConaill MA 1946 Studies in the mechanics of the synovial joints: displacement on articular surfaces and significance of saddle joints. *Irish J Med Sci* 6:223-235

MacConaill MA 1946 Studies in mechanics of synovial joints: hinge joints and nature of intra-articular displacements. *Irish J Med Sci* 6:620-626

MacConaill MA 1953 Movements of bone and joints. Significance of shape. *J Bone Joint Surg* 35B:290-297

MacConaill MA 1966 The geometry and algebra of articular kinematics. *Biomed Eng* 1:205-212

MacConaill MA 1966 *Studies on the anatomy and function of bone and joints.* F. Gaynor Evans (ed). Springer, New York

MacConaill MA, Basmajian JV 1969 *Muscle and movements: a basis for human kinesiology.* Williams & Wilkins, Baltimore

MacConaill MA, Barnett CH, Davies DV 1962 *Synovial joints.* Longmans, London

Marey J 1891 *La Machine animale.* Alcan, Paris

Moreaux A 1959 *Anatomie artistique de l'homme.* Maloine, Paris

Netter FH 2004 *Atlas d'anatomie humaine.* Masson, Paris

Occam (*or* Okham) William of (English Franciscan monk and scholastic philosopher, 1280-1349) *The principle of economy*: see the Internet

Özkaya N, Nordin M 1999 *Fundamentals of biomechanics,* 2nd edn. Springer, New York

Poirier P, Charpy A 1926 *Traité d'anatomie humaine.* Masson, Paris

Poitout DG 2004 *Biomechanics and biomaterials in orthopedics.* Springer, London

Rasch PJ, Burke RK 1971 *Kinesiology and applied anatomy. The science of human movement.* Lea & Febiger, Philadelphia

Riemann, Georg Friedrich Bernhard (German mathematician, 1826-1866) *La géométrie non euclidienne* (on Codman's paradox): see the Internet

Roud A 1913 *Mécanique des articulations et des muscles de l'homme.* F Rouge, Librairie de l'Université, Lausane

Rouvière H 2003 *Anatomie humaine descriptive et topographique.* Masson, Paris

Roy-Camille R, Roy-Camille M, Demeulenaere C 1970 Ostéosynthèse du rachis dorsal, lombaire et lombo-sacré par plaques métalliques vissées dans les pédicules vertébraux et les apophyses articulaires. *Presse Med* 78:1447

Roy-Camille R, Saillant G, Mazel Ch 1986 Internal fixation of the lumbar spine with pedicle screw plating. *Clin Orthop* 203:7-17

Saillant G 1979 Étude anatomique des pédicules vertébraux. Applications chirurgicales. *Rev Chir Orthop* 62(2):151

Sobotta J 1977 *Atlas d'anatomie humaine: nomenclature anatomique internationale.* Maloine, Paris

Steindler A 1964 *Kinesiology of the human body.* C.C. Thomas, Springfield

Strasser H 1917 *Lehrbuch der Muskel und Gelenkemechanik.* Springer, Berlin

Testut L 1893 *Traité d'anatomie humaine.* Doin, Paris

Thill E, Thomas R 2000 *L'Éducateur sportif.* Vigot, Paris

Von Recklinghausen H 1920 *Gliedermechanik und Lähmungsprostesen.* Springer, Berlin

Index

Mechanical model of the cervical spine

This model is the **exact functional equivalent of the mechanical model** described on pages 224-231 of this volume. With some attention and patience you can build it starting from the structures included in Plate 1. To avoid damaging this book you should use a photocopy of the whole page, preferably enlarged by 50% to make the task easier. Then use a sheet of carbon paper (which may be difficult to find since the disappearance of typewriters) in order to transfer carefully the diagrams onto the cardboard. Avoid using Bristol board, which is too flimsy, and select a sheet of cardboard that is at least 0.3-0.5 mm thick, e.g. photographic paper used for colour printers. This cardboard must be rigid enough for you to be able to assemble and use the model. If you cannot find carbon paper, use a 3B lead pencil to blacken the back of the photocopy of the plate. This is equivalent to a carbon paper, and you need only go over the drawings to reproduce them on the cardboard underneath.

The model consists of **six pieces** that must be cut out:

- **the head A**, with its hinges y (dot-dash line) and z (dashed line), which you must remember to fold in opposite directions (see later)
- **the intermediate piece B**, linking the head to the spinal column and containing a shaded area on the front and a corresponding area on the back for gluing
- **the cervical spine proper C**, which also contains a shaded area to be glued to the intermediate piece
- **the base of the model D**, with its three shaded areas for gluing and two sets of slits (S1-S3)
- **the tunnel strap E**, with its two areas for gluing in the back and two dashed lines to be folded in opposite directions
- **the support strap F**, with at one end a shaded tab for gluing on the front and at the other an unshaded tab.

Cut-out procedure

After cutting out the pieces you must **prepare the folding lines** (indicated by dashed lines) while **following these instructions.** First use a craft knife, a scalpel or a razorblade to **cut partially into the cardboard to one-third of its depth.** Make the cuts **on the front of the cardboard along the dashed folding lines** and on the back along the dot-dash folding lines so that you can bend the first type of fold backwards and the second type forwards. To make this easier, draw the folding lines on the back of the cardboard. You can mark the ends of these lines by piercing through the cardboard with the **point of a compass.** For piece C, representing the cervical spine, make the oblique cuts along the dashed lines **on both sides** of the cardboard to allow bending on both sides. To avoid weakening the cardboard you should make the cut on the back about 1 mm above the cut on the front.

You must **pierce the holes without fail before assembly,** since by making them after assembly you are likely to weaken the model. If you do not have a punch, you must try to make the holes as neat as possible in order to allow easy passage of the elastic bands later. The holes in two corresponding pieces must **coincide exactly.**

Assembly

1. Assembly of the base

Important: Keep the glued surfaces in place until they are dry; use paper clips or electricians' crocodile clips.

- Start with the **tunnel strap E.** Plate 2 shows how it can be folded into an omega Ω after cuts are made on both sides of the cardboard (Fig. I).
- Glue its two 'paws' on to the two small **shaded areas** on D so as to form a small tunnel for the flap of F (Fig. II).
- With a blade, cut a **horizontal slit as marked on F.**
- Make a cut on the front of the cardboard for the central fold (dashed line) and on the back for the lateral tabs (dot-dash lines) in order to fold F like an accordion (Fig. II).
- Glue the **shaded 'paw'** of F on to the large shaded area of the base (Fig. III).
- When the pieces are tightly glued together, thread the **other 'paw'** of F into **the bridge strap E** to complete the construction of the base (Fig. IV). The base is now set up.

2. Assembly of the cervical spine

- Fold the central flap in A twice, i.e. backwards along z (dotted line) and upwards along y (dot-dash line) to form a **solid right angle.**
- Glue the surface of the strip below axis y to the shaded area on the upper surface of B, making sure that the holes (c and a′) coincide (Fig. IV).
- When these are tightly glued together, fold the shaded area of C backwards and glue it to the lower surface of the unshaded part of B (Fig. IV). Once more make sure that the holes (c and c′) coincide.

3. Assembly of the model

- Check the notch at the base of C and slip it into the slit of F in order to fix C to the base (Fig. V).
- To strengthen the structure you can also place a matchstick or a toothpick through the hole k in C just under the arch of F.
- The model should now stand up straight; however, once you have made the oblique folds in C (dotted lines) more pliable, it will tend to bend to one side. This instability of the model reflects perfectly the **natural instability of the cervical spine**, which is steadied by **muscular stays.**

Stabilizing the model

To keep the model straight you **need to stabilize it with narrow strips of elastic**.

This operation calls for meticulousness and patience. An elastic band can be secured at one end by a knot made on top of one of the already punched holes and at the other end by passing it through **one of the slits already pierced by scissors** (S1-S3) at the margin of the base, where you can **control the tension in the band by securing it tightly**.

These elastic tighteners fall into **two groups** (Figs VI and VII):

Group 1 These tighteners (solid and dashed blue lines) control the upper part of the model corresponding to the suboccipital spine with **three axes** represented by **three hinges**, i.e. the **vertical hinge** for rotation of the head, the **horizontal hinge** for flexion/extension and the **sagittal hinge** for lateral flexion. They include the following:

- Elastic 1 is attached above hole a, passes through hole a' and is secured at the slit S4 at the right degree of tension. It controls **flexion/extension** of the head.
- Elastic 2 passes through hole b' and is fixed by knots at holes c' and b with the right degree of tension in it. It controls **rotation** of the head.
- Elastic 3 is knotted at each end above holes c and c' after passing through the slit S5. By pulling on it on either side of the slit you can control **lateral flexion** of the head.
- Elastic 4 is secured like elastic 3, but it is a little longer since it passes through slit S6. It controls at the same time lateral flexion of the head and the **stability of the upper part of the spine.**

Group 2 These tighteners (solid orange lines) control the **lower cervical spine** with elastics 5 and 6, corresponding to the **scalene muscles**; they keep the cervical spine straight along its vertical axis:

- Elastic 5 is knotted at hole e and is secured at the right degree of tension in the two slits S1 on of the base.

- Elastic 6 is knotted at hole d and is secured at the right degree of tension in slits S2 on the base.
- Elastic 7 is knotted at holes c and c' and is secured in slits S3. It is the lateral stabilizer of the model.

As you adjust these various elastic bands you come to realize how **unstable** is the cervical spine, which needs to be steadied by the muscular stays and how any change in one of the stays will alter the balance of the whole structure. This means that the cervical spine is an **integrated functional unit** and **any disruption in one of its anatomical components will have an impact on the whole structure.**

Once the elastics are adjusted, you can **experiment** with the various movements of the cervical spine.

First **move the lower cervical spine** at its oblique hinges (dashed lines) and you will clearly observe its **stereotypical movement of lateral flexion-rotation**. From this position you can use the suboccipital system, which is equivalent to a tri-axial synovial joint, to impart to the head the following **corrective movements:**

- **rotation in the direction of motion**, which brings to completion the lateral flexion of the head
- **lateral flexion** in the direction opposite to that of motion associated with **rotation** on the side of motion; this results in pure rotation of the head.

If you hold the base and the head (A) firmly, you will be able to perform the **movement of the Balinese dancer**, i.e. a translational movement on either side of its axis of symmetry. This movement, which is **unnatural**, requires countercompensations that you can figure out for yourself.

Your efforts to build this model will be rewarded and you will be able to perform all possible types of movement and compensations in the cervical spine.

Take heart!

Plate I

Plate II

I

a

b

c

II

III

IV

V

Plate III

VII

VI